SUBTEXT

SUBTEXT

SUBTEXT

KATE MARLEY

Published by Accent Press Ltd – 2010

ISBN 9781907016455

Printed and bound in the UK

Cover design by
Zipline Creative

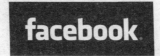

Prologue

YOU MIGHT HAVE SLIPPED outside to take a call on your phone when you first saw us, or, if you're so inclined, have been finishing a crafty cigarette before heading back into the warmth of the bar. Either way, we draw your attention, standing in a gap between the buildings, across the street and along a little way from where you're standing.

Don't get me wrong, that's not to say I'm especially stunning, or that he is. We look like any other couple on a night out, neither unusually dressed nor especially loud, not even remarkable in our unremarkableness. But there's an intensity of something brewing between us that stops you short, making you look in spite of the fact it's bloody cold and you were actually getting ready to go back inside and rejoin your friends.

His hand is clenched around my upper arm, in a grip so visibly tight even from this distance that you wonder fleetingly if it's going to bruise. He has pushed me up against the wall, his other hand tangled in my hair holding me in place, so when I try and look away – for help? – I can't.

He isn't particularly big or broad, in fact you'd probably describe him as nondescript if you were to bother describing him at all. But there's something about him, something about us, that makes you wonder for a minute if everything is all right. I can't take my eyes off him and the obvious depth of my awe means for a second you can't either, staring at him intently trying to see what I see. And then he tugs on my hair, pulling my head closer to his in a vicious movement that makes you instinctively step a bit closer to intervene, before those stories in the papers about good Samaritans meeting sticky ends flood your brain and pull you up short.

Closer now, you can hear him talking to me. Not the full sentences – you aren't that close – but enough words for you to get a sense. For these are evocative words. Vicious words. Ugly words that make you think perhaps you really might have to step in at any moment if this escalates further.

Slut. Cunt. Whore.

You look to my face, so close to his, and see fury glittering in my eyes. You don't see me speak, because I don't. I'm biting my lip, as if I'm restraining the urge to respond, but I remain silent. His hand tangles tighter in my hair, and I wince as my scalp stings but otherwise I stand there, not passive exactly – you can feel the effort it is taking for me not to move as if it were a tangible thing – but certainly self-controlled, weathering the verbal onslaught.

Then a pause. He is waiting for a response. You move closer. If someone asked you'd say it was to check I was all right, but in your heart you know that actually it's curiosity, pure and simple. There is something feral, primal, about the dynamic between us that draws you closer even as it almost repulses you. Almost. You want to know how I am going to respond, what happens next. There is something dark and yet compelling about it that means while normally you'd be horrified instead you're intrigued.

You watch me gulp. Run a tongue along my bottom lip to moisten it before trying to speak. Starting a sentence, tailing off, eyes flickering down to break his gaze as I whisper my response.

You can't hear me. But you can hear him. 'Louder.'

I'm blushing now. There are tears in my eyes, but you can't tell if they are of anguish or of fury.

My voice is clearer, even loud on the night air. My tone is defiant yet the flush, both on my cheeks and running along the collarbone visible under my open jacket, betray an embarrassment I can't hide.

'I am a slut, sir. I have been wet all evening thinking about you fucking me and I would be very grateful if we could go home now and do that. Please.'

My defiance cracks by the last word, which comes out as a soft plea.

He runs a finger idly along the edge of my shirt – low cut enough that there is a hint of cleavage but not exactly slutty – and I shiver. He starts to speak and the tone of his voice makes you restrain the urge to shiver too.

'That almost sounded like begging. Are you begging, slut?'

You see me start to nod, but get pulled up short by his hand in my hair. Instead I swallow quickly, shut my eyes for a second and answer.

'Yes.' A pause, turning into lengthening silence. A breath which might almost be a quiet sigh. 'Sir.'

His finger is still running along the curve of my breasts as he speaks.

'You look like you'd do pretty much anything right now to be able to come. Would you? Do anything?'

I stay silent. My expression is wary, which surprises you bearing in mind the obvious desperation in my voice. You wonder what "anything" has encompassed in the

3

past, what it's going to mean now.

'Will you get down on your knees and suck my cock? Right here?'

Neither of us speak for long moments. He removes his hands from my hair, steps away a little. Waiting. The noise of a car door slamming a distance away makes me flinch, and I shift to glance nervously up and down the street. I see you. For a second we make eye contact, my gaze widening with shock and shame before I look back at him. He is smiling. Utterly still.

I make a sound in the back of my throat, half whimper, half plea and swallow hard, gesturing around vaguely. 'Now? Wouldn't you rather we –'

His fingers press against my still-moving lips. He is smiling, almost indulgently. But his voice is firm. Imperious even.

'Now.'

I cast the quickest glance possible your way. You don't know it, but in my head I'm playing a very adult version of a childish game – if I don't look at you directly you're not actually there to witness my humiliation, can't see it because I can't see you.

I gesture nervously in your general direction. 'But it's still quite early, there are people walking –'

'Now.'

You are transfixed watching the battling emotions flit across my face. Embarrassment. Desperation. Anger. Resignation. Several times I open my mouth to speak, think better of it and remain silent. Through it all he just stands there. Watching me intently. As intently as you are.

Finally, face crimson, I bend at the knees and drop down to the wet cobbled stones in front of him. My head is bowed. My hair falling in front of my face makes it hard to tell, but you think you can see tears glistening on my cheeks in the light of the street lamp.

For a few seconds I just kneel there, unmoving. Then you watch me take a deep, steadying, breath. I square my shoulders, look up and reach for him. But as my shaking hands make contact with his belt buckle, he stops me, patting me softly on the head the way you would a loyal pet.

'Good girl. I know how difficult that was. Now get up and let's go home and finish there. It's a bit cold for playing outside tonight.'

His grip is solicitous as he helps me to my feet. We walk past you, arm in arm. He smiles. Nods. You half nod back before you catch yourself and wonder what on earth you're doing. I am looking studiously at the ground, my head down.

You can see I am shaking. But what you can't see is how aroused this whole experience has made me. How hard my nipples are in the confines of my bra. How my trembling is as much from the adrenaline high of everything that has just played out in front of you as it is the cold and humiliation. How I thrive on this. How it completes me in a way I can't fully explain. How I hate it yet love it. Yearn for it. Crave it.

You can't see any of that. All you can see is a trembling woman with dirty knees, walking away on wobbly legs.

This is my story.

Chapter One

THE FIRST THING TO say is that I am not a pervert. Well, no more than anyone else. Someone coming to my flat would be more struck by the piles of washing up in the sink than my dungeon – not least because the cost of living in the city is such that I'm lucky to have been able to find somewhere with a living room which I could rent alone within my budget. Let's just say a dungeon wasn't really an option.

I am neither a doormat nor a simpleton. I don't yearn to spend my day baking while someone hunts and gathers for me and I keep the home fires burning, which is just as well as apart from a decent Sunday roast I'm a bit of a crap cook. I also don't look like Maggie Gyllenhaal from *Secretary*. Alas.

I just happen to be, at points when the urge takes me and I have someone I trust to play with, a submissive. Not that it shows to people who don't know me. It's just one facet of my personality, one of the plethora of character elements that make me, well, me – coexisting with my love of strawberries, compulsion to continue arguing stubbornly even when I know I'm wrong and tendency to heap scorn on ninety-nine per cent of television programmes and yet become obsessive about the other one per cent to a level that frightens even me.

I work as a journalist on a small local newspaper. I

love my job, and – not that it should really need to be said – being submissive doesn't impact on my work. Frankly if it did I'd get lumbered with tea-making and picture stories about infant school book weeks, which really is a fate worse than death. Also, newsrooms are bantery places. It's a dog-eat-dog world and you need to give as good as you get. I do.

I consider myself a feminist. I'm certainly independent. Capable. In control. To some that might seem incongruous with the choices I make sexually, some of the things that get me off. For a while it seemed jarring to me. In fact, sometimes it still does, but I've come to the conclusion that frankly there are more important things to worry about. I'm a grown woman of mostly sound mind. If I want to relinquish my personal control to someone I trust for them to lead us somewhere which proves thrilling and hot for both of us, then as long as I'm not doing it somewhere where I'm frightening small children or animals I think that's my right. I take responsibility for my actions and those choices.

It has taken a while for me to get to this stage, though. I would, if the word hadn't been appropriated by reality television into something that sounds both nausea-inducing and in need of a soft rock video montage, go so far as to say it's been a bit of a journey, which is really how this book came about. This isn't a manifesto or a how-to book, although I like to think if you're into this kind of thing and wanting to explore you might get some ideas. It's just what happened to me, how I discovered and explored this side of myself, my experiences, my thoughts. Ask another sub their thoughts and what being submissive means to them and you'll get a whole other different book, probably with significantly less sarcasm.

Looking back on it now my submissive tendencies

started young, although I wouldn't have called them that then. I just knew there were certain things that made me tingle, that I would find myself thinking about wistfully without ever really being able to put my finger on why.

I've always been into myths and legends, and growing up Robin Hood was a favourite. I watched the films, the TV show – we'll overlook the most recent incarnations before I start gnashing my teeth – and read all the books I could lay my hands on, fictional and historical. But through every medium I had a difficult time with Maid Marion. I hated that she was continually getting into peril for stupid reasons and then having to be rescued. That she didn't fight, wasn't even given the relative dignity of being a bona fide sidekick and seemed to spend most of her time patching up the wounds of the Merry Men and looking pensively into the middle distance as they disappeared off for adventure.

Despite that, my favourite parts of those stories involved her in the very peril I scorned her for. When she had been captured – as the inevitable bait in a trap to catch Robin Hood, seemingly her major purpose in life – her defiance of Guy of Gisburne and the Sheriff of Nottingham captured my imagination. She would be held in some dank dungeony place, with the pictures often showing her tied or in chains. Powerless. But she would be unbowed, dignified in her indignity, and somehow that struck a chord with me, made my heart race. You know how, when you're a kid and something you read or watch catches your imagination so deeply that you are transported into it, it's you in that moment, living it, feeling it? (Actually, I say "when you're a kid", don't judge me but I still feel that now when I read or watch something amazing, it just happens less often). Well all the scenes I replayed in my mind with me in the lead role were the scenes of Lady Marion. Even if she was a bit rubbish and I tended to gloss over the dull stuff after Robin saved her and she got to go back to the camp and resume tending the fire. Those were the stories I used to think about lying in bed at night.

Well at least until I discovered porn.

When I was about fourteen there was a brouhaha about a magazine that gave away an erotic book aimed at women with their issue one month. Lots of talk of moral decay and the like meant that I spent weeks desperate to get hold of a copy, in part because I'd started to suspect I was dirtier than my school friends, or at least dirtier than they dared to admit aloud they were. Even aside from getting to see exactly how scandalous this stuff was, it could, I reasoned to myself, act as a kind of smut barometer.

Except there was a problem.

My next door neighbour worked in the only newsagent big enough to sell the magazine in our village, and there was no way she'd let me buy it. So one afternoon I took a different bus home that took me to the nearest big town and bought the magazine there, hands clammy, still wearing my school uniform, terrified at any moment that the uninterested woman behind the counter would realise I was underage and shamelessly buying what the *Daily Mail* had described as utter filth and demand I give it back before I ended up inadvertently corrupted for ever. She didn't. I stuffed it in my rucksack and, my heart still pounding, walked the two miles home to explain to my mum I was late because of hockey practice.

Looking back at that book, now so well thumbed that the pages have started to fall out although I can't bear to chuck it away, the scandal and outrage at the time seems laughable. But reading it then, it was a revelation. My favourite chapters still have the tops of the pages folded over for ease of finding. One particular section involved a feisty yet vulnerable woman having a row with a man who she clearly fancied but also found herself continually clashing with. She ended up tied to a tree with ivy (I know, it's a bit lame, but go with it, it was special Greek ivy, which may have heretofore unknown bondage qualities) while he did whatever he wanted to her – running his hands over her body, viciously kissing her, verbally abusing her. She stood there, aroused in spite of herself and he made her come, all without her being able to do anything but rest her head against the tree and moan out her pleasure. It sounds quite cheesy indeed now, almost Mills and Boon-esque, but at the time it struck a chord with me. Suddenly that was what I was replaying in my head as I lay in bed at night, now accompanied by a hand between my legs rubbing myself to bring about blissful sleep.

Of course, there comes a time in every girl's life where actual boys overtake both books and the Guys of Gisburne of our imaginations (I was never really the Robin sort). My first serious boyfriend, older but not wiser, initially seemed somehow to pick up on signals I didn't even know I was giving out. Unlike other boys I'd kissed he'd hold my head firmly in place, my ponytail twisted around his hand as we kissed goodnight and I loved it. I loved feeling under his power, immobile as our tongues duelled.

I used to daydream about the possibilities of those kisses, what they could be a prelude to, the hint they gave of a different side to him, a side the world didn't see; although I felt it, as if that side of him was calling to a complementary side of me. And then one night he bit my lower lip, so hard I whimpered into his mouth in a kind of

11

surprised pleasure. Instantly he broke away, nearly taking a clump of my hair with him in his haste, and apologised for hurting me. It felt awkward to explain that actually I'd liked it, so I accepted his apology, said it didn't matter, and went indoors disappointed, with my nipples erect and my knickers moist.

I still didn't really know the significance of that exciting me, all I knew is that nice girls didn't get off on such things, or if they did they certainly didn't talk about it. So I didn't. I went about my life, going through all the usual milestones, losing my virginity, going to university, with all the hedonistic freedom that it offered, including my first sexual experience with a woman.

Nothing really changed until I met Nick, who, at least, if he didn't exactly lead me astray (by this point I was capable of coming up with enough dodgy thoughts of my own), certainly opened the door to a new world. A world I hadn't understood my longing to visit, even if I had been vaguely aware of its existence.

My first taste of kink, like many people's, I suppose, came from a good sound spanking.

I like to think I have a fairly good imagination. I certainly have a (and I say this not so much with pride but as a statement of fact) very dirty mind which means I'm more than happy to come up with alternate uses for innocent-looking objects. That, combined with my financial priorities at university – books and beer, not necessarily in that order – meant a lot of my favourite sex toys were reused household items.

So I liked to think there wasn't anything amongst the stuff in my room which could be picked up and used for nefarious purposes against me that I hadn't already thought of (and quite possibly played with), which was why the hairbrush was such a big surprise.

I have very thick hair and a lot of it. Not in a werewoman way, but in a way which means, first thing in the morning, when I'm warm and sleep-flushed, my sartorial style often owes a little something to the wild woman of Borneo.

As it often does after a good fucking.

At that point though, we hadn't even got that far. We'd been kissing for what felt like hours, the kisses of two people wanting to tease out the tension a little longer, each kiss and movement of the mouth a prelude and a promise to something more. Finally we surfaced in an unspoken agreement to move on, my face raw from his goatee and my nipples visible through my top, he with an obvious bulge in his trousers. As we broke apart he untangled his hands from my hair, with some difficulty.

As I tried to finger comb it into some semblance of order he pulled my hand away and kissed each digit, his dimple flashing as he gave me a smile which was on the very edge of wolfish. 'Forget it. We're just going to muss it up again anyway. And it's OK. I like to see you mussed.'

I stuck my tongue out at him as I began unbuttoning my shirt. 'I can't help my hair. And, anyway, yours is looking pretty unkempt at the moment too.' I gestured vaguely over my shoulder, gently mocking. 'There's a brush over there you can use if you need to.'

Nick's hair was at least as unruly – even before I had anchored my fingers in it while we kissed. It was significantly shorter than mine, but the front continually fell in front of his eyes, causing him to do an unconscious ruffling thing to pull it away from his head when he was saying something important. I found it, and him, adorable.

I'd met him in the library during my third year of uni,

which makes us both sound more diligent than we actually were. He was a politics student, kind, funny and good company but very serious. He was sexy in a brooding and slightly geeky way; we had been dating casually for a while, although as he was an American graduate student on a term's exchange at my college neither of us had any plans for it to be a serious thing. He was the most considerate lover I'd had, though, which meant I was definitely making the most of him while he was around. However, I would never in a million years have picked him out as being into anything remotely kinky, which made what happened next my first lesson on not making assumptions about people.

I turned away and pulled down my trousers, bending down to pick them up from the floor where they were pooled around my feet. That was when he hit me.

It was the sound that did it I think. That and the fact that I wasn't expecting it. When someone smacks you so hard on the arse that the room echoes with the noise of it and it's totally unexpected, it hurts. Even if in the back of your mind you're thinking 'that was only one bloody slap for goodness' sake' you can't quite resist the urge to rub your arse. Or I couldn't, at least.

I turned round, my fingers still on my stinging arse, to see his eyes wide and innocent, his smile wider as he waved the paddle brush in front of me. 'You said I could use it.'

Feeling like I was standing on the edge of something amazing that I had been waiting for years to experience, I smiled back at him, screwing up my courage, giving him the permission he was hinting at. 'You're right. I did.'

Serious hair needs a serious hairbrush and that is what it was. As he pulled my knickers down, pulling me across his lap and started smacking me with it, the noise

14

ricocheted across the room, leaving me worried about what on earth my flatmate would think from next door, at least until he'd been going for a few seconds, after which point I really didn't give a toss.

I had often wondered what a good hard spanking would feel like. But in a million years I would never have expected it to feel like *this*.

It hurt, obviously. A lot more than I was expecting – you can tell I'm of the generation that didn't get corporal punishment in school. The air whooshed from my lungs with each impact for the first few hits, and all I could think of was how much it hurt – definitely not the sexy paddling of my secret fantasies. In a panicked inner monologue I was trying to decide whether to put a stop to it or just try and withstand it until he moved on when, suddenly, the sensation changed, blossomed almost. It still hurt, but the sting of my arse melted to a pleasurable ache in the seconds after the impact and, as the adrenaline pumped through me, suddenly even the pain of the initial hits was blurring with the warmth of the pleasure I was getting out of it.

He'd started on my left cheek, hitting me in a regular rhythm until my heart was practically beating in time with his tempo, my body responding to the slaps of him beating me. He varied where the brush landed until the whole of my arse cheek was warm and I was squirming across his lap in an incoherent bundle of nerve endings. In that moment my world was him and me, the stinging warmth of my arse, the wetness between my legs, the feeling of his cock hard against my thigh as I wriggled against him. If he'd asked me what I wanted him to do, if I'd been capable of forming words, I'd have been begging him to stop as the pain was on the edge of becoming too much. But at the same time the warmth between my legs meant I knew with utter certainty that, if he had stopped, within a few seconds I'd have been pleading for him to continue. I didn't actually get the choice, which is just as well as, by that point, there was no way I was capable of speech.

He switched cheeks, and the process began again. But as I tried to temper my reaction to the pain, I felt a finger slide along my cunt lips, and easily – so easily that I was glad I was facing away so he couldn't see the sudden blush on my face – he pushed inside me.

By this time I was practically writhing on his lap, my breathing heavy, tears behind my closed eyes. He didn't hold back on hitting my arse with the brush, and, as I turned to look up at him, I saw the flush of exertion and excitement on his cheeks, and an expression that made me whimper. He looked so sexy. The look in his eyes, the way he held his head, had changed him from the Nick I had previously known. I couldn't take my eyes off him. He was power. Control. He made me feel warm and cold and excited and nervous and like the whole world was being turned upside down and all I could do was hold on for the ride and trust him to lead me through it.

As our eyes met it was like a spell was broken. We were both more than ready to fuck, and, while he wasn't going to leave a job half done, the last three smacks with the brush were quick, albeit hard enough that I gasped at the pain. My mind was spinning; I couldn't breathe enough in between hits to prepare for them. I rode the waves of pain as best I could and was still gasping as he manoeuvred me on to all fours ready for – *please please please* – us to fuck.

My cunt was filled and I moaned in relief, and then in confusion when it became apparent that it wasn't his cock filling me. I turned round, eyes blinking and trying to focus, to see him smiling at me again and holding the brush from the wrong end so he could show me my juices glistening on the handle. He tucked a strand of hair behind his ear as his dimple flashed again, a glimpse of playful Nick. 'Sorry, I couldn't resist.'

I harrumphed and opened my mouth to answer, only to be stopped when he pushed himself deep inside me. As we fucked, me grinding down on him as feverishly as he pushed himself up into my wetness, the pain from the already forming bruising of my arse, the stinging heat of it, was, with every thrust, a harsh reminder of the punishment.

He leant forward, frigging my clit as our movements got more frenzied and desperate, both of us close to coming. Just at the point where I felt I couldn't go any harder, or take any other stimulus anywhere, he ran the brush, metal bristles side down, along the full length of my still throbbing arse. It was like running needles across my flesh. I couldn't help it, I screamed. If I could I would have begged him to stop, purely because the sheer force of feeling was so great I thought I was going to faint. But as fast as my brain shorted out, saying I couldn't cope and it was all too much, my orgasm came, and with it the flood of warmth that makes me want to curl up and rest for ten minutes, before doing it all over again.

We lay there, tangled in the sheets, the sweat from our exertions drying as our breathing returned to normal. And as I looked at him, his eyes closed and his long eyelashes making him look angelic, it was almost impossible to reconcile him with the man whose punishment I would be feeling every time I sat for days. I couldn't figure out how I'd never thought of a hairbrush that way before. Suffice to say, I haven't overlooked its possibilities again.

I also never looked at Nick in quite the same way

again. As we both came down from our adrenaline highs there was a moment of embarrassment. He ran a gentle hand over my arse, assessing the damage and enquiring politely whether I was in a lot of pain. In a way that seems very British, somehow, I said I was fine thank you and then we fell silent. I think he felt disconcerted by how much he enjoyed punishing me – one of our earliest drunken discussions in the uni bar was about how he respected women more than I did as I believed porn was acceptable if the women involved were happy to do it, while he adamantly (and, I suggested, judgementally) did not – and looking back I wonder if he made a discovery about himself that night as he wielded the hairbrush.

He certainly helped fit one of the earliest pieces of the puzzle for me. By the time he was preparing to go back to the States a few weeks later my arse had become intimately acquainted with that brush – and his hand – several more times, including one notable occasion when he got so aroused punishing me he came across my buttocks and then rubbed his spunk into my still-stinging bum. We had embarked on the beginning of a dance of dominance and submission but neither of us seemed quite sure what the next step was. Although during our last night together I had a glimpse of what might have been, and even now – years on and with the experiences I've had since – I still think it had the possibility of being really something special.

I'm not really a fan of outfits. I've been known to dig out my old grey gym knickers and netball skirt for school disco nights; I've been persuaded to turn up to the occasional fancy dress party. I have even, on one memorable occasion, dressed as a nurse, after a special request from my then boyfriend, and I had to restrain

18

myself from giggling while administering his bed-bath with extras. I'm just too self-conscious to do outfits. I feel ridiculous and when you feel ridiculous it's hard to feel sexy.

But the corset was different.

As I kicked my shoes off, chucked my keys down and headed into my bedroom to get ready for my farewell dinner with Nick, I found the box on the bed. It was one of those boxes so understated and discreet that despite its lack of label it screamed 'ridiculously expensive boutique'. As I fingered the cream ribbon bisecting it, my flatmate plonked herself down on the stool in front of my dressing table, mug of tea in hand, waiting to see its secrets. Apparently Nick had brought it round for me half an hour before as a goodbye present, telling her he didn't want me lugging it home from the restaurant.

Being both impatient and a big kid at heart when it comes to giving and receiving presents, there was no hope of me waiting till after the date to open it. And, as I rationalised to Mel, he obviously wouldn't mind, or he wouldn't have brought it round.

When I first opened the box all I could see was tissue paper. And then as I pulled back the folds and pulled out the gorgeous corset nestled within I took a little breath of wonder. It was a rich vivid green. The kind of green that reminds you of lush countryside and summer and fucking outside amid the smell of fresh-cut grass and sunshine.

'Kate, it's beautiful. Are you going to wear it tonight?'

It was a gift as surprising as it was stunning. Being a tomboy at heart it was not the kind of thing I would normally have chosen to wear and it seemed an unusually tender gift for him to give me.

As my fingers caressed the delicately finished edge I looked over at Mel.

'How could I not?'

As it was only 40 minutes until I was due to leave to meet him, there wasn't much time for fussing. I picked a pair of tailored trousers which I knew flattered my arse, hopped in the shower and was back and ready to be laced up within 20 minutes.

The bodice was rigid and boned, with black ribbons running through eyelets down the back. Since there was no way I was going to be able to do it up myself, Mel came in and, once I'd slipped it on and tried to adjust myself into it as much as possible, began the process of lacing me up. It was a very long process.

As her nimble fingers pulled the laces tight between each individual set of eyelets I felt my body – and my mindset – alter. My posture changed, my curves seemed to swell and contract into an hourglass figure unlike anything I could ever have imagined possible. My breathing became shallow, my ability to move was curtailed and my busy day, the hassles of the journey home, even the bitter-sweetness of the night ahead all faded away. All I could feel was nerve endings tingling, and a roaring sound in my head. My nipples, pressed tight into the boned panels, were taut and aching and suddenly hard-wired to my cunt. I could feel myself getting wet just standing in the thing, and momentarily rued the fact I had gone for trousers, since the seam between my legs was only going to add to the distracting sensations.

There was no time to change, even if I'd wanted to. Fortunately I'd sorted out my make-up and hair beforehand, as Mel had tied the laces up with an efficiency that meant movement was seriously hampered. It had pulled me in and up in such a way that my breasts were spilling over the top of the bodice, pale and soft against the green. Suddenly I had a cleavage which was distracting me, let alone anyone who would be face-on to it. I made a mental note to throw on a jacket I could do up to the neck for the tube journey.

As Mel clasped my waist and turned me round to get the full view, she unconsciously ran a gentle finger along the edge of the bodice above one of my tits, only catching herself when I shivered slightly at the additional sensation. She blushed slightly and we both laughed.

'Sorry, it's the velvet. It's screaming out to be stroked.'

By the end of the night it wasn't the only thing doing so.

The journey to the restaurant was interesting. We met at Oxford Circus tube, and, although he could see I was wearing it, Nick didn't make any comment about my outfit as we walked to the restaurant and were shown to our table. But as I tried to find a way to settle myself comfortably in the seat he stifled a smile at my dawning realisation that the corset wasn't as innocuous as it might have looked. It was a beautiful and yet fiendish form of restraint.

Dinner was lovely but eating too much wasn't an option. As I excused myself for a loo trip he smiled at the way I moved, my gait so different from my usual carefree, 100-mile-an-hour dash through life. My movements were careful and slow, and I felt like a different person – more aware of my femininity, aware of every nerve ending, more submissive, more demure even – and that's not something I've ever really been big on.

It was also making me feel ridiculously horny. I was fast realising that this corset was a kind of subtle bondage. Our dinner was one of the most sensual meals of my life, which is quite impressive for a small Italian restaurant with a student-friendly budget tucked behind Oxford

Street. I spent the evening aroused and desperate to go home, my skin flushed my heart thumping.

We finally went back to my place. He stripped off my trousers and knickers, tied my hands behind my back with the ribbon from the box, which I'd chucked on the floor in my haste to open it earlier, and then we fucked. He sat on the stool and I rode him, grinding myself onto him until we were both gasping.

He pulled my tits free from the constraint of the corset, but the reprieve was brief before he turned his teeth and fingers to my aching nipples. As I panted, my breathing shallow and constricted by the cruel beauty of the boning, he frigged my clit and sucked my breasts until I came, shuddering and whimpering in a hybrid of pleasure and pain.

With small tremors still reverberating through my limbs I sank to the floor and finished him off with my mouth, looking through my now wild hair into his eyes, watching him stare greedily at the vision of slutty debauchedness I presented kneeling at his feet. As he tangled his hands into my hair and fucked my mouth for the final few thrusts I sucked him deep.

We said goodbye the next day. We were both exhausted and sated; my body was covered with bruises, not only on my arse but also around my breasts and torso from Mel's enthusiastic tightening of the corset. The brush that had started it all (and which I received my hardest punishment to date with at the end of that night) went back to the States with Nick as part of his leaving present.

I've never met him again, although I often think about him. I wonder about looking him up on one of the social networking sites but then I think, well he hasn't looked for me, so maybe it's best to leave things be. I know this sounds like hippyish crap, but I do believe we meet people for a reason. Looking back on it now, what Nick and I did together was relatively tame. But it was my first taste of playing with someone who was a dominant foil to my submissiveness, who didn't judge me for what turned me on and let me see fully what did the same for him. I'll always feel gratitude for that.

He also left me the corset. I still have it. I even wear it sometimes, although it is so tainted with memories, even years later that just slipping it on and beginning to tighten it sees my juices begin to pool between my legs and my nipples harden.

The rest of my time at university passed quickly. I realised that my feelings for Nick were deeper than I had admitted to myself. Forlorn at his loss, and grappling with a dissertation and my finals, my life was all work and no play.

Even when I did find someone who might tempt me from the straight and narrow, the encounters were, in contrast, vanilla and attempts to try and make them otherwise ended in disaster. I asked one partner (Graham, Geography) to spank me while we were shagging and saw him look at me in horror before – forgive the pun – giving me a few half-arsed slaps and then resuming what he'd been doing previously, before never calling again.

When I asked coquettishly, over drinks, another prospective date (Ian, Maths) whether he fantasised about doing anything particularly kinky he blushed slightly and told me he quite fancied having sex with me while he wore my clothes. I think I managed to keep my face from betraying any horror – goodness knows I have enough unusual proclivities of my own to respond negatively to anyone else's – but I didn't end up seeing him again, funnily enough.

It's fair to say I missed Nick a lot. Although I did find it easier sitting on the wooden chairs of the lecture hall after he'd gone.

Chapter Two

I met Russell in a queue. It was a very long queue, and we were in it for a long time. When I first met him I thought he was an arse and if I'd had anywhere to escape to I would have wandered off and not spoken to him again, which with everything that's happened since would have been a real shame.

I was chatting to a friend and he interrupted. He was alone and obviously bored and I remember thinking he was rude, arrogant and clearly thought a lot of himself, although my irritation was tempered by finding him attractive. After two hours' chat – and a surprising amount of laughter – I had a grudging liking for him and when he suggested all of us exchanging numbers to go out for a beer we did so, secure in the knowledge he wasn't an axe murderer and would be good company over a drink or two.

When I gave him my details I never expected to find my wrists tied to his headboard and him looming over me with an evil half smile that made me wonder for a second just what I'd let myself in for.

We'd been fuck buddies for a while by that point, so it was inevitable we would end up having a conversation about long-term unfulfilled fantasies. But as I knocked back a glass of red, giving him a brief summary of what had happened with Nick and the experiments I'd had with internet smut, before shyly admitting I fancied unleashing my submissive side properly with some experimentation into BDSM, I really didn't see him as the one. And I wasn't even expecting him to become the one – as far as I was concerned we were having a bit of horny chat as prelude to a perfect end-of-week pick-me-up fuck. I'd come to appreciate his intelligence and his deliciously dirty mind, but little did I know I had crossed paths with someone who it would turn out was ying to my submissive yang.

He was fully clothed, which made me feel even more vulnerable as he knelt over my naked body to reach my nipple. To start with he was just playing, rubbing his fingers over and around it, watching it bud. I started to relax, my eyes drifting shut to enjoy the sensation, when he pinched it. Hard. I gasped at the sudden burst of pain and looked up to see him staring intently at my face. He released his hold for a second, but the respite was brief, as he adjusted his grip for a tighter one before beginning to pull harder, tugging my breast high.

The pain increased and my breath started to shudder. I bit my lip and arched my back to try and ease the tension, but with him kneeling across me, and my wrists tied, I couldn't move far, and having watched my writhing with amusement, a slight move of his hand meant the full bitter-sweet pleasure of pain was back a second later. My moan filled the room and all that ran through my mind was the thought 'well, it really was as arousing as I remembered', at least until the warmth of the pain in my nipple filled my mind and I wasn't thinking of much else at all.

He turned his attention to my other nipple, licking delicately round it before sucking hard and grazing it with his teeth. I bucked underneath him at the pain. If my hands were free I'd have been running my fingers through his hair, but instead all I could do while he alternated between gentleness and cruelty was clench and unclench my fingers, unsure which it was I was actually craving at that moment.

Actually, I'm lying. The pain was turning me on more than I'd expected. More than my enjoyment at being spanked by Nick had even hinted at being possible. And as Russell ran his hands down my body I shamelessly spread my legs wider so he could see the glistening proof.

He chuckled and gently ran his fingers through my wetness towards my clit. In contrast to the treatment of my nipples, his strokes were light, frustratingly so, and I lifted my hips to encourage him to push his fingers deep inside me. But as I moved, he moved away. I looked up in frustration and he raised his eyebrows at me.

I knew what he wanted, I spent a good twenty minutes blithering on about how I thought it would be sexy to have to do it. But somehow begging seemed so much easier in fantasy than in real life. I guess I'm just contrary, a typical stubborn Taurean, but having spent years dreaming of properly giving up control, when the moment came to do it, in person, with a sexy man whose mind was a mystery to me, it felt like maybe I wasn't ready to give it up just yet after all.

As the silence lengthened it became a battle of wills, which was stupid since I knew him touching me would be a victory for both of us. His hand rested gently on my mound, one of his fingers tapping gently on my clit – one, two, three times – like he was drumming his fingers on a table, while I decided what to do next. His calm infuriated me more. So I stayed silent. Definitely more stubborn than I thought I'd be, which ironically enough is a recurring theme which has got me in trouble many times in the years since.

A pause.

Russ moved his hand away and turned to face me, running a finger, slick with my juices, around my mouth. I sucked it deep, tasting myself, licking him clean, and trying to somehow reassert a semblance of control. And yes, I know that, having spent so long yearning to give it up, it sounds really contrary. As I pulled his finger deeper into my mouth, he smiled at my unspoken – and, admittedly, unsubtle – suggestion, pulled down his trousers and pulled his cock out. I strained forward, eager, and he fed himself to me. I sucked him, smiling around him as I heard him sigh his pleasure.

I've always loved giving blow-jobs – but never more so than with Russell. Even during the most vanilla of shags he seemed so in control, and I loved shaking that up a bit, seeing his reactions, hearing his breathing quicken, feeling him grow in my mouth, tasting him as he came. I may have been giving up my control, submitting to his power, but with my mouth round his cock I had a different kind of power and it made my heart sing and my cunt wet. And right then, tied down, his cock pushing between my lips as I lay on my back on his bed, that felt reassuring.

As I began to suck harder, he grabbed my hair. I moaned round his cock, glancing up to look at his face as I sucked deeper, moving eagerly, quickly, relentlessly, until his spunk slipped down the back of my throat. He sat back to regain his breath, running his hands lazily around my thighs. By then I was gagging for it. I'd learned that moving didn't work in my favour though, so I lay passive as he ran his fingertips up and down, coming closer and closer to where I was aching for him to be. If I hadn't been tied down I'd have been frigging myself senseless just to get some release, but instead I had to lie back, submit, as his finger slipped over my clit, an all too brief burst of pleasure, before going back to stroking meanderingly around my thighs.

Suddenly the whole issue of begging or not begging didn't matter. I was so desperate to come that I'd have said pretty much anything if it meant he'd let me. My hands were clenched into fists, I was biting my bottom lip and finally through a dry throat I was able to say: 'Please.'

His finger moved back to my core, gently stroking. He was definitely looking smug now. 'Please, what?'

The tone of his voice was different, darker, and it thrilled me and yet left me uncertain. This wasn't easygoing, laid-back Russell. It turned out my fuck buddy was a man of surprises. But not a man of patience.

He pinched my nipple again, twisting it viciously. Tears filled my eyes and I gasped in pain. His voice was steely, not to be disobeyed and made me even wetter, even as nervous butterflies moved in my stomach.

'Please, what?'

My brain locked. I'm someone who's never lost for words, but I had no idea what I was supposed to say and was terrified that if I got it wrong he'd draw it out even longer. Or, even worse, stop. In the end in spite of myself I went for every variation that might do it.

'Please, push your fingers inside me. Please touch me. Make me come, let me come. Please.'

As I finished on the final plea he began to frig me – strong, long strokes which I'd been yearning for for what seemed like hours. He slid two fingers inside me and began fucking me with them, rubbing, harder, faster, until I couldn't contain my cries. I shuddered, moaned, and came, pulsating around his fingers, my hands bashing against the headboard with the force of my orgasm.

As he pulled the knots so my hands fell free, he smiled. And as I rubbed my wrists I smiled back, knowing that I'd found a kindred spirit in the oddest place, that we'd be doing this again. That it was even worth begging for. What I didn't realise, not then at least, was that actually that was hardly begging at all, and only the beginning.

I am, by nature, a cynical woman. Blame it on being a journalist although, actually, I should probably admit it's a character trait that predates that. I don't believe in Santa Claus or the Easter Bunny. Which makes what happened the first time Russell took his belt to my arse even more amazing. It definitely happened, but I know it's ridiculous and it's not happened since. At the time though... Wow.

The first time he made me beg was just the start. While we were firm friends, we had no plans to date, but, in a way, that made discussing what turned us on easier – telling your boyfriend that you fantasised about him caning you until you were sobbing and then fucking you hard against the marks even as you fought to push him off could potentially be a bit awkward. But Russell listened closely to everything I said and, although I didn't realise it at the time, was mentally making notes for things to do which would make my cunt wet and my head spin.

It really started one Saturday night, with punishment for a host of spurious reasons which, if I was feeling argumentative, I would have queried. Except of course when his voice and mannerisms changed from easygoing to implacable and it became apparent exactly where we were headed I really wasn't going to quibble, especially since I ended up naked with my arse in the air, bent over the arm of his sofa.

He began with a relatively gentle spanking, which left

my arse tingling and warm. I'd learned early on that Russell was a fan of spanking, and he had soon developed a penchant for putting me over his knee to punish me while his erection grew under my squirming body, my knickers halfway down my legs; which felt somehow more embarrassing than having them taken off completely, as well as proving helpful for him hobbling me if I couldn't stop myself struggling. Previously once my arse was hot and stinging he'd push me to the floor and fuck me, his hips anchoring me hard to the floor as he pushed inside me, ensuring no relief from the rough carpet against my stinging arse, but this time things were different. He asked me a question which I didn't answer with what he deemed to be quite the correct level of respect and I heard the sound of his belt slipping through the loops of his trousers.

When you have spent so long thinking about something, fantasising about it, the prospect of actually being on the receiving end of it is terrifying. Not just because it's going to hurt and suddenly lovely, kind, just-finished-helping-me-do-the-crossword Russell has shifted into an alternate version of himself. Not just because I'm desperately trying to control my nerves, to ensure that I don't chicken out, hoping that I can withstand whatever he doles out, please him and acquit myself with courage and stoicism – ah yes, Lady Marion would be proud. Not even because, having spent the best part of a decade lying in bed at night fantasising about what it would be like for someone to give me a good old-fashioned thrashing with a belt, I'm concerned that in practice it might not be arousing and instead it might just hurt so much I would have to get him to stop and not only would that be a disappointing enactment of a long-held fantasy, but a form of surrender, failure, a defeat too far.

I turned my head, which was hanging down towards the floor, giving me a headrush to add to the dizziness of my anticipation, to see him standing in front of me, still fully dressed, holding his leather belt in his hands, pulling it, looping it, getting ready to hurt me, and the look in his eyes made my stomach lurch with the same mixture of fear and excitement you get on a rollercoaster. And then he moved behind me and all I could do was wait and try not to tremble. I didn't have long to go.

The first strike didn't hurt that much, the noise was more of a shock than the impact itself. I felt a moment of relief that actually the pain was bearable, and then he hit me twice more in quick succession and I yelped loudly – it would appear he'd not got the aim or the strength of his swing right with the first hit as it was hurting a damn sight more now.

He told me the more I yelped the harder he would hit me, so I bit my lip to try and silence myself, until I was convinced I could taste blood in my mouth. The crack of each impact on my arse sounded like a gunshot and the pain after the impact was a wave of agony. If it wasn't for the arm of the sofa under my abdomen holding me in place my legs would have buckled till I was lying on the floor in front of him. As it was, when the flick of the end of the belt curved round to catch one of my arse cheeks in a place it had hit several times before the white hot pain caused me to wobble, sliding halfway to the floor, until he grabbed a handful of my hair to encourage me – in unrelenting and rather painful fashion – to scrabble back into position.

My tiny gasps were almost sobs by the time he asked me to count the blows. The pain was so much more than I could ever have imagined, but it didn't occur to me to ask him to stop. Instead my mental focus was on withstanding the impact, stifling the moans and whimpers bubbling up into my throat with every lash, although trying to control my breathing to work through the pain must have given away how much he was hurting me if the angry red stripes on my arse, the tears streaming down my face, and my shaking legs, didn't.

After ten strokes he put his hand on my clit, frigged me hard and then pushed his fingers up inside me, laughing softly at how obviously, audibly, aroused I was.

'Oh yes. You are quite the little pain slut, aren't you, Kate?'

I shut my eyes, even as the noise of his fingers moving between my legs proved his point.

As he rubbed me and I began to moan in pleasure, he explained to me the concept of the carrot and the stick – and exactly how after my rudeness I wasn't in line for the orgasmic carrot just yet. He pushed me back up into position for punishment without removing his hand from my cunt and I felt a moment of fury at being treated like a fucking hand puppet. I could almost see his smile as I strained on tiptoe across the arm of the sofa, his fingers pushing cruelly up inside me. I counted another ten hits with the belt through my dry throat – plus 'one for luck' which I'm sure he just inflicted to amuse himself at seeing my visible relief at the end of the punishment being replaced with shuddering nerves as I waited for the final – and hardest – blow.

Before I could even gather my wits his fingers were back on my clit. He was frenetic, rubbing me so hard that even with the lubricant it was bitter-sweet pleasure. I came hard, and my legs gave out from under me, leaving me slumped across the end of the sofa. As I lay getting my breath back, my hair sticking to the sheen of sweat on my back, his voice was close to my ear.

'You have a choice. You can either get me a tissue or lick my fingers clean.'

I looked at him askance. One thing that we both found arousing, even before we realised we had the more hardcore kinks in common, was me licking my juice from his fingers after he'd made me come. Why would I want him to use a tissue? Then he showed me his hand. Turns out that the carrot and the stick game – and the most vicious scene we'd ever played and the intense orgasm it generated – had inspired female ejaculation, which was surreal and pretty bloody hilarious since I'd spent years telling everyone who'd listen it was a ridiculous myth perpetuated by porn stars.

After I'd recovered sufficiently, I knelt at his feet, sucking him until he spurted in my mouth and then slept the sleep of the exhausted, on my side because my arse had taken such a battering that even the whispering movement of a duvet on it made me wake in pain. It took days for the welts to go down and every morning, after my shower, I checked the changing colours of the bruises in the full-length mirror, prodding to see how much it hurt and smiling to myself at the same time.

Yup, I was beginning to understand the full extent of my masochistic tendencies. And in Russell I seemed to have found someone that not only recognised them too but enjoyed giving them a good workout, although I was soon to realise that actually it wasn't necessarily the pain that was the most challenging element of playing with my incongruous dom.

Chapter Three

THE DAY AFTER MY intimate introduction to his belt we headed into town for a spot of lunch and a trip to the cinema – experiencing the joys of mid-week days off when it feels like everyone else has their nose to the grindstone while you're bunking off.

We'd grabbed the papers and headed into a restaurant. As my bum hit the hard wooden bench – why are they so popular? They're horrible and the interior designer of *Wagamama* has much to answer for – I grimaced slightly. noticed and smiled but didn't say anything until the waitress had taken our order.

'Is your arse sore?'

Pride? Stubborness? An urge to wipe the undeniably sexy but still damn conceited look off his face? Probably. 'It's OK.'

'Really? You looked quite uncomfortable when you sat down.'

We shared a look that said he knew what I was thinking and I knew he knew but was going to do my best to ignore it anyway.

I didn't get much peace. We chatted about film possibilities for the afternoon, a woman at work I fancied, the latest in an ongoing love/hate saga between two mutual friends, and ate our lunches. Then once we'd finished he took a sip of his drink and looked over at me for long seconds without speaking.

'What?' I asked.

He put his drink down on the table. 'Nothing, it's just every so often you shift on that bench and when you do your face changes and I can see it hurts.' He smiled. Bastard.

I tried to act like it was completely normal to be discussing the thrashing he gave me over the remains of two club sandwiches. 'Actually I thought the cane would have been more painful. But last night –' I shifted without thinking to find a more comfortable way to sit, only becoming aware of it when I saw him smiling at me, '– well, the belt was a lot more painful. I don't know why really.' I raised my chin. 'But it doesn't hurt that much.'

He raised an eyebrow and I realised that I'd just unwittingly given him a challenge that would come back to haunt me.

'To be honest, I did hit you hard, because I knew you could take it, that you love it in fact. But I was only giving you about 75 per cent of what I could – because we were so near the wall I couldn't get as much swing as I wanted.'

My arse clenched at the thought of being beaten any harder with the belt, now an innocent fashion object round his waist once more, which I couldn't drag my eyes from.

'Of course I don't know if you'd be able to take much more. Your arse was looking pretty battered by the time I'd finished. And you could hardly stand to lean over the arm of the sofa, your legs were shaking so much. I'd have been worried except for the fact your juice was running down your thighs so I could tell exactly how much you were enjoying it. Dirty girl.'

I was lost for words. I think I may have managed a "guh", but that's about it. As I looked round the restaurant

– ladies who lunch with a gaggle of small children a table away, a couple of teenagers making a smoothie last while rummaging through a bag of purchases – I tried to regain some semblance of control and ignore the warmth pooling between my legs. It was working too, sort of, until –

'The thing with the belt I love is how it flicks round the side of your arse with each lash. I'm sure it's painful on impact but it's the last flick round the curve that seems especially harsh. The marks it leaves are great though. And I love how you shudder when I run my fingernails over them. I could wank just looking at your punished arse. Although that could leave you ultimately pretty frustrated.' He smiled in a way that showed he really didn't care and I was aiming once more for the bantering coherent-ish speech we'd been at a few short minutes ago.

'It'd be OK, I'm sure I could sort myself out if the need arose.'

Another wolfish smile. 'Ah, now there's an excuse to tie you down. Not that I really need one.'

My breath was getting ragged and I was definitely wet. I crossed my arms on the table in front of my breasts so no one could see my nipples which were, inevitably, tight in my top.

I laughed quietly, with a faint air of desperation I couldn't disguise. 'We should stop talking about this now.'

He smiled. 'Why? Are you turned on?' As if he didn't know. Except of course he did and was asking because he enjoyed seeing me blush as I answered.

My "yes" was very quiet.

'Move your arms away from your chest.'

I muttered his name, the word both a plea and exclamation of exasperation, my arms still firmly covering my now tight nipples.

Then the tide turned and his dom voice was right there, the bantering gone. "It wasn't a request, Kate."

Slowly I moved my arms away.

'Move back in the seat a little so I can see you properly.'

My face was hot as I moved back.

He laughed softly. 'That really was a little. It's OK though, it was enough.'

He stared intently at my breasts, not breaking away when the waitress came to ask if we wanted dessert. He ordered for both of us, and when she'd gone and I pointed out she'd seen him doing it he replied: 'Ah, I wasn't staring at them, I was just thinking what they'd look like naked.'

I gulped my drink. Oh, that was all right then.

As we waited for dessert, conversation reverted to the topic of Kath, the girl at work who might or might not be bi, but any hope I'd be given a chance to compose myself from the horny, wet, incoherent puddle sitting in front of him was soon extinguished. Having met her briefly he'd decided she was a switch, someone who could be either dominant or submissive, depending on who she was playing with, and began explaining to me exactly how he'd go about showing her how to "get the best" from me.

As he described tying me down, making me lick her out, showing her how to use the cane effectively on my arse and tits, making me watching them fuck, and so much more, I was beginning to move on the bench for different reasons. I was wet, horny and as I tried to eat my dessert my hand was shaking holding the spoon.

All of which he noticed, of course.

By the time we'd finished and got the bill I had no interest whatsoever in going to the cinema. I wanted to go back to his house for rampant mid-afternoon shagging.

When I told him this – OK, maybe not "told", there may have been pleading on my part, I really was very horny by this point – he smiled.

'OK. We can go back. But not yet, I have some things I want to get first.'

He could see the frustration in my face but I wasn't going to complain as I knew he'd just spin it out longer. So we paid the bill and started walking. I was wearing jeans and no knickers at Russell's request, so walking around with a seam pressed along my slit drove me crazy.

By the time we'd been into a DVD shop, two bookshops, and a supermarket I wanted to scream with frustration. He wasn't even buying anything. I'd given up even pretending to browse and was just focused on not embarrassing myself in public either by begging him to take me home and fuck me or coming to a seam-related orgasm. Finally he walked up behind me as I stood staring vacantly at a display of magazines and slapped me hard on the arse, making me yelp and dragging me from my reverie.

'OK, I'm done. It's time to go home.'

Thank fuck.

We finally got back to the house and as soon as we got through the door I suggested a blow job. I was desperate and wanting to reassert a little control. Russell's ability to read me had left me on the back foot and I figured getting my mouth round his cock would redress the balance – blow jobs didn't make him any less in charge, but every so often he'd make a tiny noise in the back of his throat or clench and unclench his hand and I'd know that for once he was the one fighting for control and it was all because of me, a very satisfying thought. Almost as satisfying as feeling him respond to my tongue and thickening in my mouth, getting to swallow down his spunk, diligently licking him clean afterwards and the orgasm it usually guaranteed for me afterwards. Oh yes.

So on the way up the stairs I asked him if he wanted me to suck him. He smiled. 'I think I could be convinced by that. But I had something else in mind first.'

Before I could even begin to guess what he was thinking of, he'd grabbed my wrist and pulled me off-balance onto the bed. While I tried to right myself, or at least get myself in a slightly more comfortable position, he yanked my arm into the small of my back with one hand and began pulling down my trousers with the other. By the time I'd stopped struggling and become resigned to the fact I wasn't going to be able to move from the position he wanted me in he'd already grabbed the hairbrush off the side table and the sound of the first strike on my arse was echoing around the room.

The rhythm was relentless. Sometimes his punishments were light and playful but this was anything but, even though it was only a few hours after he had used his belt on me. I don't know how long it went on, I was just focused on riding the waves of pain.

By the time he paused to run his fingernails and then the bristles of the brush along the burning red marks of my arse all I knew was that my face and my cunt were both wet. He pulled me back up, running his hand along my slit as I stood in front of him on wobbling legs. Chuckling he pushed his finger into my mouth for me to suck it clean, pointing out that for all my tears and whimpers as he punished me I was now tasting the proof I enjoyed being treated that way. I blushed as I licked my juice from him, hating his smugness – and the fact he was right.

Once his finger was clean he ordered me to strip and

then when I was naked pushed me to my knees. He took one of my tight nipples in each hand and pinched them, mauling them between his fingers until I was biting my lip to avoid crying out. Finally he tired of the game and pulled his cock free. I set on it like I was starving.

But he wanted control of everything. He tangled his fingers fully into my hair and began fucking my face at his speed, indifferent to my stinging scalp and struggle to breathe as he dragged me up and down his cock. Then suddenly, his hands tightened and he pulled me away from his crotch.

'I'm not coming in your mouth.' I looked up at him in confusion. 'I'm going to come on your tits. And as soon as I have you're going to lie back on the bed and I am going to do what you've been gagging for me to do all day. I'm going to make you come.

'But there are rules. A good cumslut doesn't spill any. If any of my spunk drips off you and hits the bed I'm going to stop what I'm doing, immediately. I'll make you get dressed and you can go home wet, whimpering and unsatisfied. Do you understand?'

I nodded, watching intently as he ran his hand up and down his cock. And then he came, in long milky spurts across my breasts and stomach. Taking a step back he smiled at me. 'Well what are you waiting for?'

I sank carefully to the bed, gasping at the pain of lying on my still throbbing arse.

'Does it hurt?'

I nodded.

He smiled again as he grabbed my arms at the wrist and moved them to make me hold the headboard of his bed.

'Shame. Just remember what happens if you spill any.' He ran a hand along my inner thigh and I trembled. 'I

41

have a feeling you'd rather not go home frustrated.'

Then he started fingering me and I was lost. He ran his fingers along my slit and then pushed them deep up inside me. He finger fucked me relentlessly, while grinding my clit with his thumb. I was moaning and squirming in pleasure but every movement caused zinging pain as my arse brushed against the sheet. The sensations merged until the pain and the pleasure and the humiliation and the sheer sexiness of it was all one, my loud moans shattering the silence.

Russell stopped for a moment, taking a step back to look down at me, staring intently. I blushed, wondering what kind of picture I must make lying there covered in spunk, legs spread, cunt dripping and begging to come. Then I realised he was checking whether I had let any of his spunk drip off me as I writhed.

I was desperate. I went to move my hands, to catch the dripping spunk with my fingers but his tut as I shifted halted me in my tracks. For a split second we looked at each other, my eyes no doubt narrowing as I realised exactly what this meant, while his twinkled, his lips widening into a smirk at my reaction when I realised what I needed to do if I wanted to ensure my orgasm.

Who am I kidding? There were no ifs involved. Even as my brain processed what he was expecting, and wondered if I would do it, I was already moving my body. I twisted awkwardly on the bed, each brush of the bedding against my welts making me suck air in through my teeth. One particularly forceful movement, made as I saw a droplet of spunk moving inexorably round the curve of my hip in a way which filled me with panic, saw me bashing the side of my arse against the bed hard enough that I whimpered. Still I kept moving, while he watched my inevitably futile attempt to thwart gravity.

Finally, he took pity on me. 'If you're having trouble, you can use your hands.'

Thank fuck. Desperately I ran my hands along my rib cage and the sides of my breasts to catch his cum, greedily licking my fingers clean before putting my hands back on my now glistening and also flushed chest. Feeding myself his spunk in sluttish fashion seemed to please him as – thank goodness – he started pounding his fingers inside me again.

It was like swimming against conflicting currents. The relentless frigging, fingers pounding into my cunt, the still raw pain of my arse pushing against the bed as I writhed. Feeling so many different sensations, all the while trying desperately to ensure I didn't spill a drop of his spunk meant that it took me a long time to orgasm despite my desperation. Suffice to say, my cunt was aching by the time the need to orgasm overcame any fears of failing at my role of cumslut.

When I did come I came hard, my moans and eventual screams ringing loud in my ears. I trembled for a long time afterwards with the intensity of it all. He stroked my shoulder as the shudders subsided and as I looked over at his still fully clothed body I was reminded that even I could underestimate him sometimes. It was also one of the most memorable shopping trips I've ever been on, which is pretty bloody amazing when I didn't actually buy anything.

Chapter Four

THE PROBLEM WITH BEING a masochist is that, when it comes down to it, if your dominant isn't an utter sadist then punishments in the usual sense of the word don't really work as a deterrent.

After all, the ebb and flow of pain as a cane lashes the curve of my arse where it meets the top of my thigh makes me wet. Drugs aren't my thing but the high I get when the adrenaline is thrumming through my body is a legal (and free!) equivalent to that rush. It stays with me for at least as long as the marks do, occasionally rushing to the forefront of my mind during the days after a session, catching me unawares as I grind through my vanilla, professional day, a flash of memory making my nipples hard, my body ache, my eyes glitter in a way that might make my colleagues wonder exactly what I am thinking about in that moment where I seem elsewhere.

All in all, hardly a punishment.

Of course what this means, if you're playing with a dominant as evil as Russell, is that he watches to find out the thing that you don't find sexy. The thing you do at his behest while gritting your teeth, as an act of pure submission. The thing you hate, and do just to please, usually while pretending it doesn't bother you because you know if he realised just how much you hated it he'd make you do it more just because he could. The thing you don't want to do. Aren't sure you can do. Which leaves you with stormy eyes, flushed with anger and humiliation, wishing you could tell him to fuck off but knowing that you can't because in spite of yourself you crave this even if you can't explain why.

For me, that is the foot thing.

There are many amazing things about Russ, both in terms of character and appearance. He is intelligent, funny, has the most expressive, gorgeous blue eyes, a dirty smile and the ability to keep me on the back foot like no one else I have ever met. Personally and sexually he challenges me in a way that makes life just seem that bit sharper, colours a bit brighter. However, and there really is no getting round this, he has feet like a hobbit. And a hobbit after a hard day's gambolling about the Shire at that. While I can see why some people fetishise them and, well, each to their own, feet really aren't my thing anyway, but Russell's feet specifically, well they make me shudder, and not in a good way. And he knows this.

We'd been out with a group of friends and messing about, play-fighting and being silly. Our D/s relationship remained to the outside world a subtle and sporadic one, a dom/sub with benefits if you like, and our mutual friends knew nothing about it. However, when I tapped him on the head with the rolled-up magazine extolling the virtues of the latest releases showing at the cinema and caught his nose hard enough to make his eyes water things shifted. I dug a tissue out of my handbag, while apologising for my cack-handedness. Taking it from my hand he smiled as he wiped his eyes. 'It's OK,' he said, loudly enough for everyone to hear, before adding 'I'll punish you for it properly later,' in a voice meant just for me

Suffice to say I spent a great part of the film wondering exactly what that meant. His tone wasn't unduly pissed off but it promised something out of the ordinary, so not his hand. The cane? The whip? His belt? A ruler? Would he punish me, fuck me until he came and then leave me unsatisfied – something he had done one memorable and hideously frustrating sleepless night a few months before where I been left with my hands tied behind my back and his spunk dripping from my desperate hole while he slept like a baby? God I hoped not. I was definitely up for something more satisfyingly fun.

In the end he chose something that made a night of frustration look like a walk in the park. In fact I think I'd rather have had a month of frustration. And I'm not really the chaste type.

I was on my knees, naked, on his bed when he explained to me what was going to happen. He was stroking the small of my back, running a leisurely finger up and down my spine in a way that – paired with the chill in the room and fierce anticipation – meant I was already distracted enough that for one hopeful minute I thought I'd misheard him. Definite wishful thinking.

'Do you understand?' he asked.

I stayed silent, hoping he'd actually say he'd changed his mind and instead was going to beat me until I cried and then fuck my bruised and throbbing arse without lube in recompense. That'd hurt like hell and definitely count as a punishment as I can't take him up my arse easily at the best of times. Would that count? Could I suggest it? Would that count as topping from the bottom?

He stopped stroking my back and instead pinched one of my nipples. Hard.

'I said, do you understand?'

I swallowed hard, and – unable to speak – nodded. What is it they say? You can understand but not comprehend? That was me. He had just asked me to do something that I just didn't think I could do. I didn't want to do it. The thought of doing it made me feel sick with humiliation and anger – and also a bit queasy. I'd seen him strip his boots and socks off earlier. This was not in any way alluring to me. Even the usual submissive satisfaction I get from knowing I'm pleasing someone by demeaning myself wasn't enough to make this seem in any way sexy. At all.

He moved and began pulling down his trousers. 'Well move over then. You can kiss your way down. Acclimatise yourself as it were.' The amusement in his voice was audible and it made me furious. He knew he had asked me to do something that every fibre of my being was saying I wouldn't, couldn't, do, and he was settling down against the pillow, arms behind his head watching with a smile as I tried to process it. 'Why don't you start by running your tongue along my cock?'

OK. This I could do. This I liked to do. Great. I shuffled round on the bed to get into position. He was already hard, but as I began gently licking my way up his shaft he grew further, his cock pushing into my face, almost as demanding as its owner. I lapped at his cock, diligent and focused, running my mouth round the head, losing myself in something I enjoy. But suddenly I was dragged back to reality. Literally. Tangling his hands in my hair he pulled me up so abruptly a strand of saliva stretched from my lips to the head of his cock and then broke before I could catch my breath and swallow it back.

'Very nice, but that's enough of that.' He patted my head in the way you'd stroke a pet. 'Now why don't you move down and kiss and lick my balls for a little while?'

Obediently I pushed my face fully into his groin. I suddenly had a flashback to the first time he told me to do this, and how I flushed scarlet with embarrassment and hesitated at doing something so obviously meant to demean me. As I gently sucked his balls, one at a time, into the wet warmth of my mouth, his penis pushing against my cheek, I wondered what had happened to me. How did I go from tentative embarrassment to happy, even greedy, obedience? In a few months' time how much further would my boundaries have moved? How was he able to move me past my limits with such ease?

There wasn't time for self-analysis though, as he ordered to kiss my way down his inner thighs, past his knees and shins and to the top of his feet. I did so, my kisses getting faster and lighter the further down I got in spite of my fears of admonishment. All too soon I was face to toes with his hobbity feet, the room completely silent as he waited. He was insouciant, everything about him screaming confidence that I would do what I'd been told to do eventually. I felt him shift behind me, moving position to better see the war going on in my head and on my face. He misses nothing.

I could have got up and left. I could have told him to fuck off. If I'd made enough of a fuss he wouldn't have made me do it. Probably. But somewhere along the way stubborn pride and a small corner of my brain was telling me I could do this. I should do this. Even that it's sexy to do it – after all submission isn't really submission if you only obey the stuff you like to do. It was a very small part of my brain and as I got closer to his feet it shrank further. I lowered my head to his feet. *I can do this. It'd please him if I do this. If I get it over with quickly we'll move on to something else and it'll be sexy as hell.* I closed my eyes – *do his feet actually smell? Am I imagining it because I can't see them?* – and moved in even closer but I couldn't quite bring myself to take the final step. I took a couple of deep breaths and tried again. Still no good.

My lips were dry, my mind racing. *I can do this*, I thought to myself. If I did it quickly he wouldn't realise how much it was bothering me.

'Did I tell you to breathe on my toes?'

He knew how much it was bothering me. Blatantly. My voice was small. 'No.'

'Well, what are you waiting for? Go on.'

Tentatively I shifted slightly on the bed and leant down to kiss his little toe. It was a feather-light kiss, I licked my suddenly parched lips and pushed my face back down, in opposition to every screaming instinct. He made a small murmur of pleasure as I connected with his toes again and I knew it was about my submission to his will rather than the sensation of my mouth on his foot. I could almost see him smiling behind me and it made me furious, at him, at myself and the part of me that craves this even while bridling at my own, at least partially self-inflicted, abasement. I kissed each toe, gently and respectfully and slowly – I wasn't going to have him make me do it again – finishing with a lingering kiss on his big toe. And then I turned back to look at him, breathing heavily, my face and neck red with embarrassment. I was trying not to glare but his smirk made me think I wasn't hiding my ire especially well.

Succinctness was what is going to stop me getting into more trouble, so I went for brevity even though my tone was mutinous. 'OK?'

He smiled at me. 'Not quite yet. You've got the other foot to do. Lean over me and suck my toes.'

I turned back quickly, wanting to face his feet rather than look into his eyes, which seemed to see too much. It was as if he understood this part of my nature better than I did, leaving me scared and infuriated even while the intensity of the scene was making me wet. I veered

49

between feeling so exhilarated it felt like flying and wanting to smack him about the head for being arrogant.

I moved over, straddling his outstretched legs to get to his other foot, thinking I could endure this last bit of grovelling. Just do it, don't think about it. I started by kissing the top of his foot, before screwing up the last of my courage and finally taking several of his toes in my mouth. It actually didn't taste as bad as I expected fortunately, so I moved along his foot, sucking his big toe. Licking it. Worshipping it. My mind running a mental mantra – this will soon be over. This. Will. Soon. Be. Over.

Then unexpectedly he put his hand between my legs and I moaned around his foot in pleasure and surprise. Typically he took the opportunity to push his foot further into my mouth.

'You're very wet. Your cunt lips are puffy there's so much juice there. You're obviously enjoying something we're doing right now.'

I closed my eyes and kept sucking, my body responding as he pushed his fingers further into what was – to my shame – my dripping cunt.

The room was silent except for the sound of me sucking his toes, and his fingers leisurely frigging me. In spite of myself I was wet, horny and desperate to come, pushing back on his hand as he shoved his fingers inside me.

He chuckled. 'After all that glowering it turns out you like being made to lick and suck my feet. You actually like being treated like a slut, even in spite of yourself. Don't you, slut?'

I ignored him and his repeated use of what he mockingly calls "the s word", knowing he was trying to get a reaction. I reddened even more, but with my back to him and my hair falling in my face I knew he couldn't see it. Instead I kept licking, thinking it was probably a good idea I was effectively gagged by his foot as otherwise I'd be bound to say something that got me into more trouble. Instead I tried desperately to focus on making him so happy he'd let me move on to something else. Which is very difficult indeed when your nipples are hard, your cunt is sopping and you're so desperate to come that despite it all you'd pretty much do anything for release.

As he brushed my clit with his thumb I whimpered with excitement, so close to coming despite everything. I think that's when he came up with the idea.

'You seem to really be enjoying worshipping my feet now.' I huffed my annoyance through my nose, while pushing my tongue between his toes almost viciously. 'I think I should make you keep sucking them until you come around my hand. That would be amusing wouldn't it?'

Amusing wasn't the word. I closed my eyes, trying desperately to blink back tears of fury and humiliation, knowing that in spite of how much I hated doing this he was going to be able manipulate my body into getting the utmost pleasure from it. He upped the tempo, pushing his fingers harder and further inside me, jabbing my clit with his thumb with every thrust until my face was buried in his feet, and I was whimpering round his toes. I was going to ache tomorrow but his vicious, insistent penetration was doing its job and despite it all my orgasm built, and ebbed as he slowed things down, enjoying the power he was able to wield so effortlessly over me, before building it up again. And again.

I don't know how long I licked him, although when I came my jaw was aching and my cries were almost croaky my mouth was so dry. By the end I had no awareness of anything but his hand in my cunt and his foot in my mouth. I was a primeval bundle of nerve endings, desperate to come, willing to have any of my holes filled, however he wanted, so long as he would let that happen and give me the release I craved. I'd have begged him for it, but instead I sucked his toes into my mouth as far as I could take them, licked the sole of his foot and wordlessly showed him I'd do anything for him, even something that an hour before I'd have said with confidence was a hard limit.

I once read somewhere that the key to sexual humiliation is not about making somebody do something they don't want to do, it is about leading them to do things they secretly dream about doing. I can honestly say I had never dreamed of debasing myself in quite such a humiliating way and still blush when I think of it. At the same time, when I came around his fingers my orgasm was one of the most intense I'd had for a long time. And even as he made me lick his fingers clean of the sticky juice which proved how much I had enjoyed the unusual punishment, before pulling me down his body by my hair to suck his cock, I couldn't help wondering what it would be like to have to do it again.

Chapter Five

WORDS ARE FUNNY THINGS. I am happy to call my cunt a cunt. A cock a cock. A fuck a fuck.

When I am in my submissive headspace I will grovel, I will beg, I will say whatever it is my dominant demands of me. True, some of the words will flow freely, while others will stick in the back of my throat. Pleading for him to fuck me, punish me, use me, are all things I used to find difficult, but now – thanks mainly to Russell's obsession with making me say things I find embarrassing – I wear my submission like a badge of honour, my voice assured despite my debasement, proud and wet at pleasing him by demeaning myself. Calling him sir is harder, my voice then is quieter, and if I can get away with it I hide the humiliation I can't quite overcome behind the curtain of my hair. But even though it chafes I can do it. I do. And my submission ultimately brings great pleasure and release to us both.

But the word that grates, no matter how often it is said around me, is *slut*.

I know. It's a little word. And in BDSM terms it is not even derogatory one. I am comfortable with the dual nature of my personality, the fact that I am independent, capable and in control for most of my day, and yet crave giving power to my top for mind-blowing nights. And afternoons. Mornings too, actually. But there's something about the word slut that, even immersed in the most arousing scene, will jar me out of the moment like a needle scratching across a record. Men who like sex are studs. Women who like sex are sluts. I know this is the vanilla meaning. I know when I am kneeling naked in front of Russell, sucking greedily on his cock and he calls me his cumslut the context and thus the meaning is as different as night and day. But it doesn't stop my glaring up at him even as I suck him further into my mouth.

He laughs when he sees me bristle at it. I'm hardly a prude and there are so many other words which wider society as a whole would consider worse and which don't bother me at all, but slut is the one I hate. And he knows it, loves pushing me, making me explain to him exactly how much of a greedy, grateful, horny slut I am before he'll let me come. And while in the back of my mind there is a part of me bridling at the terminology and wishing I could tell him to fuck off, I obey. I obey in spite of every fibre of my being saying I don't need to do this, for the small voice which whispers that I do. It is not the most demeaning thing he makes me do but is one that stings most. An act of pure submission.

So when I saw the paddle I had to buy it.

Russell's birthday was looming and while I'd bought a couple of great vanilla presents I was looking for something extra. Symbolic. Special. Sexy.

I was looking at crops when I saw it, half pondering whether it was bad form to give someone a present which I was going to get at least as much pleasure from as he would. It was on the end of the shelf, beautifully boxed, and in the split second after I realised exactly what it was I felt a flutter in the pit of my stomach.

SLUT.

Well actually TULS, cut into 12 inches of vicious-looking black leather attached to a sturdy handle.

I couldn't even look directly at it. I stared at the toys next to it, behind it, sneaking little glances. I knew he'd love it. Love marking me with it. But the thought of walking around with that word emblazoned across my arse like a brand made me shiver in revulsion. It was perfect. But I hated it. And I knew he'd love that even more.

I stood in front of the shelf for a good ten minutes until a saleswoman came over to ask if I needed any help, presumably fearful I was a demented potential shoplifter. Her approach was the impetus I needed. I reassured her I was fine, grabbed the box – heavier than I anticipated – and almost ran to the till to pay. I'd even stopped blushing by the time I was halfway home.

In the ten days between buying the paddle and his birthday I thought about it constantly, the carrier bag a permanent reminder on my desk. Half a dozen times I decided against giving it to him, not sure I'd be able to withstand the inevitably intense scene when he finally wielded it. But in the end, I had to wrap it up. I knew he'd love it. And I could withstand this. Right? I had time to get over it. Really. It'd be fine. Probably.

His eyes sparkled when I gave it to him. His fingers traced the stitching, flexing it and swiping the air in front of me in a way which made me restrain a shudder. He watched my reactions closely, and I did everything I could not to show him how much it bothered me.

Of course he knew how much it bothered me.

I'd got myself so wound up thinking about what it would be like to be on the receiving end of it that when he smiled and thanked me and put it on the mantelpiece it felt like an anticlimax. Then he started stroking my breasts, moved lower, and I got distracted with other things.

It stayed there for two weeks and two days, not that I was counting. Every time I walked into the room and saw it I felt a flutter in my stomach. I dreaded the thought of being punished with it but part of me wondered how I would respond. Would I be able to withstand it physically? How long would the marks last?

It was a Saturday night when I found out. We'd had a very lovely fuck earlier in the evening and crashed out pretty much instantaneously. I woke from an odd dream and then watched the red illuminated clock change for more than hour courtesy of the kind of insomnia which leaves you feeling convinced that you're the only person in the world awake and incapable of switching off. In the end, I decided an orgasm was the only way to get back to sleep. So I shuffled away from him, put my hand between my legs and began frigging myself.

It was a utilitarian wank, all about the release and, hopefully, the sleep that would come afterwards. My strokes were assured, my fingers moistening my clit with juice, making me slippery so the delicious friction would bring the orgasm I so desperately needed. I was quiet, close to coming and utterly focused, which is why when he spoke from the darkness it made me jump.

'What are you doing?'

My hand stopped abruptly between my legs. Ooops. Belatedly it occurred to me he'd probably find this bad form.

'I couldn't sleep.' My voice was croaky.

'I gathered that.' He was amused but his voice had the tone I jokingly refer to as his dom voice – although only when we're not actually playing as when we are I wouldn't dare. 'What are you doing?'

Suddenly I was very glad for the darkness. It's easier

to pretend indifference at being caught red-handed when you don't have to look anyone in the eye. 'I was having a wank. I couldn't sleep and I thought a quick orgasm would help me –'

I stopped talking as he moved across the bed to spoon behind me, his hand clamping around my wrist, still nestled – albeit now unmoving – between my legs. The warm breath of his tut tickled my ear as he pulled my hand away, making me shiver against him.

'So, just two hours after I give you what, if your moans were anything to go by, was a very intense, very pleasurable orgasm, you're greedy for another one already?'

I shook my head. 'It's not like that, it's just –'

He pulled my hand up to my mouth, effectively silencing me with my own sticky fingers.

'I think it's best you stay quiet for a moment now. Don't you?'

Russell's tone was dangerous and made me wetter but a little fearful. I stayed quiet and still, not even risking a nod as I didn't want to do anything to displease him further. My nipples were hard and my body was trying to process the fact that I had been so close to orgasm and yet apparently was going without for now.

'You are a greedy slut.' I could see where this was going and my heart was already starting to race. 'You woke me up with your bouncing because you're so horny you can't wait a few short hours before you get to come again.' I wanted to argue but I knew if I did it was just going to make things worse. 'You deserve punishment. Don't you?'

I was still silent, even in the face of the direct question. I knew what was going to happen now and part of me was thinking I was knackered and not ready for the inevitable intensity, that all I wanted was to go to sleep. But I didn't dare say that so I remained quiet. Until he pinched my nipple. Hard. I gasped at the unexpected pain.

'Don't you?'

I hate it when he does this. The act of submission is one thing, but admitting that I need this, yearn for it even, always makes me blush. Which of course he knows. I tried not to sounded huffy as I responded, 'Yes.'

He slapped my breast. 'Some respect now might save you some pain later.'

I tried to restrain my tone. 'I'm sorry. Yes. You're right, I deserve punishment. Sir.' I hoped the afterthought would work in my favour although I didn't hold out much hope.

He was stroking my bare breast, running his fingers round in a very distracting circle. In spite of the tension running through my body I started to relax into the movement, enjoying the sensation, which made what he said next even more of a wrench.

'Go downstairs and get the paddle. Now.'

I was up, across the room and halfway down the stairs before my brain really began to process what this meant. The paddle. The. Paddle. Shit. Could I endure this? Suddenly I really wasn't sure, and I was hardly filled with confidence to start with. I was going to be better prepared, not groggy from lack of sleep, sexually frustrated and with my head elsewhere.

I picked it up with shaking hands and headed back upstairs, mindful that keeping him waiting was just going to make it worse. Taking a couple of deep breaths outside the bedroom door, I pulled together my tattered courage. But before my hand could connect with the handle the door was pulled open and bright light flooded my eyes, leaving me half-blinded and disoriented.

By the time my eyes had adjusted he had plucked the paddle from my hands and manoeuvred me across the room to the bed. I knelt on all fours, waiting nervously for what happened next, suddenly wishing I slept in something more than a pair of knickers.

I was staring intently at the sheet trying to prepare myself for what was to come, which would have been easier if I'd had any idea exactly what that was. He stroked my arse through my knickers, and the touch made me flinch. He laughed as I tried to regain some composure. His hand moved round.

'Your knickers are so wet I can actually see how much of a slut you are. You've stained them with your juice.'

I closed my eyes. He stroked me through the fabric of my knickers and I bit back a moan of pleasure, my body crying out for the orgasm it was so close to getting just a few short minutes before. As he ran his fingers up and down my slit, pushing the sodden material into my wetness, my breathing got harsh. I was so close to coming my legs started to buckle. I was suddenly hopeful – was he going to let me come after all?

Of course not. Wishful thinking. He stopped and I tried not to sigh in frustration. He moved up the bed and pushed his finger into my mouth. I blushed but sucked it deep, licking myself off him. He chuckled at my eagerness.

'You are a slut. We both know it and now I'm going to mark you in a way that anyone who sees you will know it too.'

He pulled his finger away abruptly and moved behind me, pulling my knickers down to bare my arse. I had spent so long worrying about how this would work that I was already trembling, trying desperately to stay in position and not give away the extent of my fear. I was mentally kicking myself for buying him the paddle, the idea of it was all well and good but the idea of walking around with SLUT emblazoned across my arse in purple bruises repulsed me. What was I thinking? What if I really couldn't do this and this was the first time I'd have to use my safe word?

My rising panic meant I heard the first strike before I even felt him move behind me. It sounded like a gunshot and made me jump. For a split second I didn't feel anything, I actually thought he'd missed. And then the pain, God the pain took my breath away. I gasped. I may have cried out. Tears filled my eyes. He might have asked me if I was OK then. To be honest I'm not sure. There was a noise like rushing waves in my head, I couldn't really deal with anything, see anything, feel anything, except for that noise – and the pain where the paddle had connected. It hurt much more than I'd expected it to. More than his belt or the cane. I realised the full impact of what I'd given him.

The next blow came before I had time to blink away the tears from the first. I was trying to control my breathing, trying not to cry. I wanted to be able to withstand it, was definitely too proud to say I needed to stop. So I sucked in gasps of air and felt the tears running down my cheeks from behind my closed eyes as I tried to work through the pain of blow after blow.

After maybe a dozen blows he stopped. I tried to pull myself together, brought myself back to the present, was aware of him moving behind me. As I cowered slightly, anticipating more punishment he moved his hand to my arse, stroking the punished cheek, even the relatively gentle touch leaving me quivering. I felt him move closer to see his handiwork, tracing the marks he'd inflicted on my pale flesh, like a painter looking at his canvas.

'Hmmm. I need to hit you harder I think. And make sure the strike connects squarely or I won't get the full effect. I think I might have to practice on one cheek to ensure I'm doing it right, and then when I feel ready I'll give you one last massive crack across the other one which should see you properly marked. What do you think?'

I tried not to shudder and closed my eyes so he couldn't see they were once more filled with tears. 'I think it's entirely up to you, Sir.'

I could hear the laugh in his voice as he patted me on the head. 'Good answer, my slut.'

He picked up the paddle again and I steeled myself for more pain, but instead he ran it up between my legs. I bit back a moan of embarrassment – it slid easily along my pussy, betraying exactly how turned on I was. I could almost see his smile as he moved the paddle round in front of me.

'Kiss it and thank me for giving you the punishment you seem to be enjoying so much.'

I brought my mouth to the leather, now glistening with my juice. My voice was small and I could bring myself to say nothing more than the barest minimum his order allowed. 'Thank you for punishing me. I'm sorry I woke you up.'

He began again.

I wish I could say that when it started again I withstood the punishment better. But the tears still flowed, although in spite of myself my cunt juices did too. Eventually, by the time my arse felt like it was glowing with the agony, he stopped. I felt light-headed with relief, until I realised what this meant.

He let the tension lengthen before he gave me the final blow, on my as-yet-unblemished cheek. I was trembling at the prospect of it and when it finally connected and the noise reverberated about the room I cried out, my legs and arms buckling underneath me. He had put all his weight into it, swung hard, and it caught me perfectly across the vulnerable stripe of skin where my bum met my thigh. I was sobbing, in pain but also in relief that I had withstood the punishment. He stroked my back, making soothing noises, telling me how I had pleased him by being brave, and how beautiful my arse looked, all red and hot.

Then he pulled me onto my back and gave me the kind of fucking which I normally yearn for, fast, hard, vicious, filling me up. Except of course under the circumstances it was just another torturous pleasure – every movement of my arse against the sheet made me cringe in pain as did his hands pinching my arse as he pushed himself deeply into me, pain tingeing the pleasure of each thrust.

Eventually I came, my cunt spasming around his cock, my cries of pleasure overshadowing the previous cries of pain. He spunked inside me, pulled out and then made me lick him clean and we fell asleep again, with me finally getting the sleep I craved.

My right arse cheek was a mess of bruises for about a week afterwards. My left was pale and pristine in comparison, except for the word SLUT emblazoned across it like a brand, which meant I had to take special care in the changing room at the gym.

I still hate the word slut, but unfortunately Russell loves it and he loved that bloody paddle. For ages afterwards he ensured that I was marked somewhere every time we played, whether it was my arse, my inner thighs – which bruise a lot easier and which, as he had to punish me with my legs spread, tended to show in embarrassing detail exactly how wet his punishments left me – and on one notable occasion a breast.

When I see that paddle my heart starts beating faster; my body reacts in a way that proves that I am indeed a slut for the punishment – and pleasure – that it can inflict, although saying it out loud remains almost more than I can bear. They say a picture paints a thousand words though, and if you see my body once he's finished playing with me then I don't need to say anything at all.

Chapter Six

OVER THE MONTHS RUSSELL and I kept playing. He kept pushing my boundaries, introducing me to new things. But then, as we got closer to the end of the year things slowed down a little.

Working in newspapers means Christmas and New Year is a busy and hideous time. While the paper's pagination gets smaller so the amount of news we have to write gets less, no one wants to work longer than necessary, and with schools closed, your local MP more often than not nowhere to be seen and businesses away for a break, it gets harder to actually find stories. Combined with the fact that early deadlines and all those bank holidays mean you're effectively writing two papers at once, filling them with the least lame features you can come up with and the much-loathed Review of the Year when all you want to do is finish early and go to the pub, all in all it makes for a pretty stressful and annoying time.

By the time I've finished up at work and headed home for Noel en famille I'm usually ready for a rest, which is a bummer really, as a few days in close confinement with my nearest and dearest is many, many things, but restful is not one of them. After a lot of food, some great presents and a few exchanged glances with my siblings wondering when exactly we began parenting our parents, I was ready for a holiday from my holiday. And that was when

Russell invited me to come and stay at his place for a while in the lull between Christmas and New Year.

Honestly, the idea of spending five days lounging around his house fussing his dog, reading, watching his big screen TV while he was at work (oh yes, he was even more unfestive than me), catching up on some reading and eating Quality Street – plus some inevitably stress-relieving sex – sounded brilliant to me, and I was in the car as fast as I could explain a hastily made-up work emergency, pack my stuff and kiss the family goodbye. I know, I'm a bad daughter.

When I arrived we hugged hello – we didn't tend to kiss, it felt wrong and too relationshippy somehow, which makes us both sound worryingly like prostitutes although it made sense to us – but as soon as I curled into him, relaxing into his familiar scent, he pulled away. Without speaking he pushed me to the floor, kicking the front door shut as he moved, undoing his fly and pulling out his cock.

His hands in my hair pulled me into position, I opened my mouth, and suddenly the thought of nativity play write-ups, parental spats and anything other than the taste of his cock were far from my mind.

He moved to lean against the front door, and I crawled with him, unwilling and (technically, since his hands were in my hair dragging me along) unable to let him out of my mouth. As I sucked my way up and down his length, enjoying his reactions, he came hard, hot spurts coating the back of my throat in a way that made me think he was looking forward to burning off some festive-season steam too. All too soon his breathing slowed and he pulled out of my mouth.

'That was great.'

I smiled at him as he zipped himself away and helped

me up, pleased and aroused at how we – apparently – weren't wasting any time getting started on the amazing sex portion of the break.

He slapped my arse. 'Come on, let's go get some lunch.'

Oh. OK.

I was wet and my nipples were visible through my top, but I could see the glint of humour in his eyes and I wasn't going to give him the satisfaction of seeing how much I wanted to come. I could wait. I'm fairly patient. OK, who am I kidding, I'm not. But what's a couple of hours between friends?

The rest of the day passed pleasantly. We went into town and looked at the sales, and I bought books and a handbag which I loved so much I could barely restrain my glee. We had lunch, went to the cinema, walked the dog, crunching along in the frost, and generally it was wonderful, restful and everything that that time between Christmas and New Year should be – all with the additional sexual tension of my awareness of the possibilities of what would happen when we got back to his house.

And then we did get back to his house. Drank tea. Watched telly. Cooked some supper. By the time we headed up to bed my patience had pretty much faltered. As we snuggled into bed he kissed me on the forehead. And then went to sleep.

Brilliant.

After the 'waking him wanking' debacle of a few weeks before there was no way I was going to risk that, so I lay quietly in bed, watching a chink of street light reflecting on the wall and listening to his soft, rested breathing, restraining the urge to smother him with a pillow. Finally I dropped off to sleep, my final thought being "tomorrow morning".

I woke up to feel Russell's erection pressing against my elbow. Hoo-blimmin-rah. Being the antithesis of a morning person there are very few things which will cause me to smile early in the day but this was definitely one of them. I rubbed him tentatively, trying to ascertain how awake he was.

'Good morning. Is there something in particular I can help you with?' His voice was wry although a good indication he was actually awake, was which was pleasing all things considered.

'Good morning. There might be something I'm in the market for.'

His chuckle vibrated his chest under my cheek. 'I can tell. I get the feeling you're a bit horny this morning.'

There really wasn't any way to deny this, so I didn't.

'Why don't you put your lips round my cock then?'

I didn't need asking twice, and turned round to lean over, licking his tempting tip before beginning to suck him properly.

He lay back, doing very little but moaning gently when my tongue touched a spot which felt especially good. I enjoyed having control of the pace and took the opportunity to tease a little. As he began to buck in my mouth I pulled back and licked and sucked his balls for a while, something he loves but which wasn't going to be enough to make him come just yet. I half expected him to complain, but – for once – he seemed happy to let me play, although he began stroking the curve of my arse, before running his fingers along the edge of my knickers. I felt myself get wetter, desperate for him to move his hand just the tiniest way, to slip in under the fabric and begin to finger me. It seemed he was good at teasing too.

Little did I realise how good.

As he pushed the gusset of my knickers into my cunt I moaned round his cock, a wordless plea for him to stop playing with me. He ignored me, though, tracing my slit up and down the outside of my knickers until I was, admittedly rather unsubtly, pushing myself down on his hand to try and get him to give me the friction I needed.

In the end, I broke away from his cock for a second.

'Please, can you just touch me? Properly?'

He laughed, and kept on with his torturous almost-stroking. 'You are desperate this morning, aren't you, poor slut?'

I managed to withhold any response to his use of the 's' word, I was so desperate to come, although I couldn't hide the frustration in my voice. 'Well you did get to come yesterday. I didn't, remember.'

He laughed again, the kind of laugh that makes my stomach dance. 'You're quite right. And you will get to come eventually, when I'm ready for you to. In the meantime I suggest you go back to doing what you were doing.'

I harrumphed quietly to myself and obeyed. If he wanted a blow job I was going to give him the best damn blow job he'd ever had and then he was going to make me come.

I sucked him to the best of my ability. I used every trick I knew about his body, did all the things I know he loves, from gently stroking his balls and then kissing them to licking the length of his cock and then breathing on the wetness to make him tingle. I worshipped him. His cock was the focus of my world, and I was going to make him come and it was going to be great and then I was going to get my orgasm. 'Cause, well, while it's not all about me, a woman has needs.

Suddenly his hand was pinching at my hip as he held me and his spunk was sliding down my throat. I let him rest for a moment in my mouth before licking him gently clean as he had trained me. And then he started to move. To get up.

I couldn't actually form words but there was a kind of grumbling noise in the back of my throat that I couldn't stop.

'What? I'm going to make us some coffee.'

'But you said –'

'I know, I said you'd eventually get to come. And you will. But not this morning.'

Don't get angry Kate. It'll just last longer if you make a fuss. Then I had a thought.

'Can't I just –?'

'No. You can't. I'll tell you when. For now you wait.' He tweaked my nipple, which felt like it was hard-wired to my cunt. 'Now get up. Come on. If you're lucky I'll make breakfast.'

I got up. Grumpy.

Now the first thing to bear in mind is yes, I could have had a wank myself. But, well, what's the point of that? He obviously had something he was plotting and, well, only submitting for the bits you want to do is pointless really. I wanted to prove I could wait, was curious as to what he had in mind for later when he would let me come. And I was stubborn. I know, I hide it well.

And so, after a breakfast that normally would have left me completely satisfied, the day unfolded. We pottered around. I did some writing and played some online poker, we walked the dog, I cooked a massive roast, we watched some DVDs, argued about the news. And through it all I didn't think at all about the fact I wanted to orgasm. OK, that might be a slight lie. Mainly I thought about not showing how much I wanted an orgasm and, for the most part, I think I managed it, except perhaps for the odd moments Russell brushed my arse or the side of my breast accidentally. Actually I wasn't sure it was accidentally, although I didn't want to draw his attention to it in case it was and I sounded like I was hyper-sensitive about it. My nipples were aching most of the day. But I absolutely was not going to show it. No way. Ha. That'd teach him.

I was fast realising I wasn't the orgasm denial type. Now this wasn't a decision I had come to lightly. If the first night had been difficult, and the morning after set me up for a day of distraction, then that night – a lengthy blow job with me knelt on the floor between his legs while he watched the news and played with my hair like I was his pet, followed by him coming across my naked breasts and me going to sleep horny and cumsplattered – made me sure.

Don't get me wrong, I am definitely not averse to some anticipation. But two days of abstinence – made worse by the fact Russell was still taking his pleasure in lots of different tempting ways – was making me seriously grumpy.

I lay in bed waiting for sleep to claim me, which – let me assure you – is actually quite difficult when, barring the odd night in a room share, I have tended to fall asleep following an orgasm either at my own hand or someone else's every night of my adult life. I was a little sticky and so frustrated I was trembling, and pondering physical violence on Russell who had tucked himself up happily and was laid on his side smiling widely at me.

'Are you OK?' he asked, knowing full well I wasn't.

'I'm fine,' I said. Usually when I say I am fine it

means I am about as unfine as it is possible for me to be without me either bursting into tears or going postal with a cricket bat.

'So this whole orgasm denial thing isn't bothering you at all?' He knows it's bothering me. But he also knows I will chew through my tongue before I admit that.

'Nah.' I am a crap liar, and I'm hoping keeping my responses short will at least make it less obvious I am lying.

'Oh good. 'Cause I thought it would be fun to explore this a bit while you're staying. I've decided, you can't come until the new year.'

As he turned over and went to sleep I felt my jaw drop open like a cartoon character. When I worked out how many days that was – four more days of torture and unreciprocated play, assuming he let me come on New Year's Day – I wanted to despair.

'If it's not bothering you so far then I'm sure you'll be fine.'

He had his back to me but I could imagine his smile anyway and it made me want to push him onto the floor. I didn't though. I didn't say anything. I didn't trust myself. And as I – finally – fell asleep my last thought was "he's joking. He's got to be joking".

He wasn't joking. By the time I had spent two days trying not to think about not orgasming I was pretty much climbing the walls. I had never really understood how fundamentally important I held being able to come whenever I wanted to and, alas, in the lines of the song I really didn't know what I'd got till it was gone. Every casual touch felt torturous. Russell brushing my elbow with his arm as he walked past me made me wet. Showering was a kind of torment with the pressure of the individual droplets of water feeling both amazing and yet, well, frankly not quite amazing enough – thus ultimately just adding to the frustration.

Over the next days Russell came up with ever more exotic ways to orgasm. The amusement he derived from me giving him blow jobs while trembling in frustration seemed to pall a little after the first half a dozen times, so he moved on to different, more fiendish, plans. I was lying on my back on the bed, gagged with knickers wet because I'd been wearing them all day, glaring up at the sexy yet irritating view of him wanking in my face when I realised: I am not a naturally abstemious type. While I wouldn't call it a hard limit – mainly because I wouldn't give Russell the satisfaction – orgasm denial was not something that I was going to be encouraging as an ongoing part of our sexual repertoire. As he came across my face and in my hair, stroking his spunk across my cheek in a gesture that would have felt tender at any other time but actually made me clamp my teeth down on the damp fabric in my mouth to try and restrain my inner fury, I made a decision that one way or another I was not waiting much longer to come.

I was also realising that the thing about Russell that made him simultaneously fun and irritating to play with was that he knew me so well, sometimes even better than I knew myself. He knew how far to push – usually just further than I would have been comfortable going – and he watched intently as I did every sexy, demeaning thing he demanded I do, to see the feelings playing across my face as I battled with whether to submit or not, secure in the knowledge that eventually I would. He could also read me better than most people I know. In part because I'm fairly forthright, although the fact I'm a terrible liar and find it difficult to hide my feelings at the best of times probably helped. So I should have known really that he was pushing me, raising the stakes. If I'd thought about it logically it made perfect sense. However, after four days without orgasm I was so distracted I had regressed to a sometime-weepy-sometime-furious bundle of nerve endings. Stringing a sentence together was difficult, something particularly embarrassing for someone whose job relied on just that. I was blunt to the point of rudeness, grumpy, and probably rotten to be around, but for all that Russell kept smiling – and was blatantly enjoying having such power to mess with my equilibrium, which just made me more cross again.

Enough was enough. By the time we'd gone to bed after another perfectly civilised evening, spent eating a leisurely supper followed by me curling up to read with the dog sat on my feet while Russ pottered on the internet and MSN, I was ready to pretty much spontaneously combust. We lay in bed together, on our backs with Russell's arm around my shoulder and his finger tracing along the curve of my neck. Despite my best efforts even this most innocuous of touches was making my breathing ragged, a fact that – of course – he was more than aware of.

'You seem a little shivery there,' he said as one particular movement strayed close to the point on my neck where – if stroked – I purr embarrassingly like a rather contented kitten. 'Are you OK?'

I'm not an idiot. I knew that he wanted to hear exactly how he was affecting me, knew that the whole pretending-everything-was-fine thing was not going to cut the mustard and that, if I wanted to come before next year, I had to explain precisely how frustrated and desperate to orgasm I was before I had any hope at all of being able to do just that. I knew that. But it still chafed. Yes, I know, I had given him that power over me. Yes, I know he knew everything I was going to say. But even so. I swallowed hard.

'I'm fine. Just a bit sensitive.'

His teeth flashed in the dim light of the room. 'Really? How come?'

Huh. It'd be so much easier to say this stuff if he wasn't so irritating in victory. And yes, I appreciate effectively this is a victory I give him, but honestly, he was three steps away from a dance of joy.

My teeth were gritted. 'You know why.' Damn. I was going for suppliant, respectful and desperate. How had two sentences made me suddenly revert to grumpy, stubborn type?

'Humour me.'

This would be why I end up reverting to type. I closed my eyes, knowing I had to do this. That this was the least that I would have to do. Suck it up. Get it over with. I sighed.

'OK. You win. You know I've been desperate to come for days, right? All I can think about is your cock in my cunt, your teeth nipping at my clit, your finger exploring my arse ...' I tailed off, losing my train of thought as my throat went suddenly dry at the thought of everything we could do, my body aching with the need for release. Suddenly aware I'd stopped talking, I cleared my throat and tried again. 'I've been trying to hide it, but we both know that I'm desperate to come, that it is all I've been thinking about for days, that my body is crying out for it–' he trailed a finger along my collarbone and a deep and involuntary shudder of need passed through my body in a way that made my cheeks heat. My voice was tremulous as I continued. 'So yes. I know we're still days way from

74

your deadline, but I thought you should know that I'm pretty much begging you. I'm sure you must realise that I'd do pretty much anything right now if you let me come.'

He chuckled. 'Anything encompasses a lot of things, Kate. And while that makes me tempted to play with you tonight and explore exactly what that means –' at this my internal monologue started singing the Hallelujah chorus '– you realise that you're agreeing to let me push you completely out of your comfort zone? How desperate are you to come? Do you really mean anything?'

The small voice in the back of my head was counselling caution but frankly the rest of my body was desperate enough to agree to anything, although I still had to swallow my nerves before I could speak. I moved my hand down to begin stroking his already semi-hard cock. 'Within the things we've agreed previously, yes, I'm agreeing to anything.'

If my life had a soundtrack, there would have been a dramatic sinister chord there, but instead Song 2 by Blur came on, which was a bit disconcerting until through my lust-addled mind I realised it was Russell's mobile phone ringtone.

And then I felt a surge of fury as he picked it up.

Don't get me wrong. I'm one of those irritating people surgically attached to their mobile, too. I like to pretend it's because I'm often on call for work, but actually it's not. I like to be in contact with people, in control if you like. My phone charges in the room where I sleep, is on my person when I'm awake, it comes on holiday with me, all that stuff.

But I like to think if I had my arm round a semi-naked woman trembling with need who had had her hand on my cock and had just told me she would do anything I wanted her to as long as I let her orgasm, and my phone rang I'd let it go to voicemail. No. Not Russell. As he picked up and started chatting to whoever it was – the Charlie Brown-style murmuring emerging sounded female, but that was all I could tell – I felt a surge of fury and another of frustration. Tears filled my eyes in overwrought, desperate annoyance as I lay against him, his free hand still tracing along the line of my shoulder even as he continued making small talk. Not only had I just begged him, something which – let's face it – still wasn't getting easier for me despite the fact he enjoyed it so much he was constantly making me do it, I had just told him I would do anything he wanted, any bloody thing and when this call had come in he'd still picked it up. The voice in my head told me to shove his arm off, get up, get my clothes on and get out, that this was not playing, this was disrespect pure and simple and a step too far, but I couldn't bring myself to move, which just made me feel weaker and more pathetic and even closer to tears.

And then he said: 'Yes, she's here right now, lying next to me, shuddering with need. As you rang she told me she'd do anything if I let her come this evening. Yep, anything. I know. Luckily I have some ideas for what anything could mean if you're interested in hearing them.'

I turned to try and look at him in the darkness. As I thought, he wasn't talking to me. At the realisation of exactly what might happen next my stomach started to lurch. Playing with other people was something we'd said we would only do after extensive prior discussion, but this, this was within the limits. Just. Although, God, the idea of anyone else hearing how desperate I was right now made me flush with shame and horror.

Yup. I'd been well and truly stitched up.

Sarah was someone Russell had been talking to for a while. She was funny, sarcastic and exactly the kind of person you could imagine having a laugh over a few drinks with in real life. While they hadn't played together in person yet, I knew Russell had been chatting to her a lot both online and on the phone, with a view to possibly meeting up to play and maybe even more. Perhaps oddly, this didn't bother me – to be honest in his time I had seen Russ date some truly rotten people, so the idea that conceivably he could end up with someone his equal and also submissive was one I welcomed. Plus I had chatted to her a fair bit and she seemed lovely, something he definitely deserved, which helped.

None of this was particularly helping with my equilibrium as Russell explained exactly what had been happening over the last few days to her in explicit detail. Listening to him explain made me feel furious and embarrassed and then – worst of all and yet so inevitably – aroused.

'… Oh yes, she was sopping. I could see the juice pretty much dripping from her cunt she was so wet. No, I didn't touch her, I just made her take her knickers off so I could gag her with them …'

I could get up and walk out.

' …It was so cute, we were in the queue at the cash point and I brushed a finger along the side of her breast. Yeah, accidentally on purpose,' I gritted my teeth, I knew it. 'You could see her nipples through her top within a second, and her eyes were all wistful. Yeah, she looks amazing – it's like she's glaring at me because she wants to murder me, but there's an undertone of lust that she can't shake that means she'll endure the rest in the hope I'll let her come …'

Actually I could just kill him now with a shoe. That worked too.

' …Yeah and she bites her lip. It's like she's trying to stop herself from speaking or whimpering or giving herself away. She doesn't realise the little half sighs she can't suppress, or the little tremors of her body. It's amazing. Right now, I control every aspect of her. Even that …'

I was furious. But I stayed. Because even while I was embarrassed and shy and unsure about what was going to happen next, even as my mind rebelled against the idea of having given him such control, let alone him bragging about it to someone else, I began to realise he was right; I knew this could be something fun, something challenging, something amazing. He was listening to her intently. And then he chuckled and I zoned back into the conversation. 'That's a pretty evil idea you know.' My stomach dropped and I huddled closer into him to try and hear what he was saying although, I realised as I moved forward, I was also rubbing myself against him desperately, my hand still on his cock, albeit shaking slightly now.

He knew what I was doing, and his hand in my hair pulling me away made it clear it wasn't going to wash. His hand tightened into a fist and I began twisting to move the way he was urging me to, to minimise the pain of my stinging scalp. He pulled me until my head was level with his crotch and then pulled me on to his cock, letting go of my hair only to put a hand over the phone's mouthpiece to say, 'Come on. Suck me. I'm discussing with Sarah how – or if – I'm going to let you come. Doing a good job is only going to work in your favour.'

As I obeyed and began sliding my lips up and down, enjoying the texture of his cock on my tongue, he moaned slightly in his throat. Sarah said something and he replied,

'Yes, she's got her mouth round my cock now. It feels amazing. She is a good cocksucker, very enthusiastic.'

I blushed in the darkness, but irritatingly felt a surge of pride in spite of myself. I tried to brush it off by focusing on the task at hand, only half listening to his conversation until I heard him say: 'So you're touching yourself now listening to this? That's very rude indeed. I don't know that you should get to come this evening either.'

I heard a plaintive tone from the other end of the phone and then – I swear – the sound of Russell's brain ticking.

'In fact, I think maybe we should make it a bit of a challenge. Maybe I'll let one of you come. Just one of you. You can each try and persuade me as best you can and the winner gets to come.'

I could hear loud disagreement from the other end of the phone, although frankly I already felt a sense of injustice and fear – I knew if there was a choice between the two of us he would be more likely to let Sarah come than me, and after all these days and the humiliation of this phone conversation, the prospect of spending another night unsatisfied was too much to bear. I began sucking his cock deeper into my mouth.

He laughed. 'Oh, Kate's pulling out all the stops. She's taking more and more of my cock into her mouth, I'm practically ball-deep now.' He murmured in pleasure and stroked my hair. 'Oh that is very good indeed. You'd have to go some to beat that.'

My heart began to beat faster at his words, and the feeling of his hand touching the curve of my arse, moving ever closer to my cunt. And then I felt his cock harden even further in my mouth. 'Oh Sarah, I do love to hear you beg.' Shit. Begging? I had no hope. While his amusement at hearing me beg meant I spent way more time doing it than I ever anticipated, the fact remained I was not a natural beggar. In fact if anything I was a grudging and slightly grumpy one. Shit.

I began gently stroking Russell's balls with my fingers while taking him further into my mouth. I'm always a keen giver of blow jobs, but even for me this was unprecedented. I could hardly breathe I was taking him so deep. His hand on my arse, stroking me gently, was both soothing and distracting. I could feel my juices pooling between my legs, dreading to think what sort of picture I must have made.

He explained to Sarah exactly what I was doing to his cock. At one point he interrupted his conversation to tap me on the arse and urge me to take his cock further into my mouth. I was so focused on doing the best I could that it was only when I heard him say: 'She is especially submissive tonight, actually. Normally I'd have expected her to disagree with some of this or at least glare as she obeyed me, but she's so desperate to come she really does seem happy to do anything,' that I zoned back into the conversation.

That's when he said again that Sarah was evil. I soon found out why. And he was right, she was.

My jaw was aching by the time he'd been on the phone for half an hour. I could hear him teasing Sarah, taunting her, making her beg, and in spite of myself it made me wet, made me wish I could hear the proof of her submission somehow in the same way she could hear mine. And boy could she hear mine.

Once Russell had finished telling her how submissive I was being he held the phone out and had me tell her. I had to explain exactly why I was so wet, what a slut I was to enjoy being treated this way. And I did it all, with a throat clogged with tears of humiliation, although I didn't think to disobey. He made me tell her that I would do anything to get to come this evening and then, once I had and he had gone back to having the phone against his ear, he clarified it further.

'She said anything. Anything. And I think she'd obey anything pretty much now. Seriously. Listen.'

He ordered me to crawl down the bed to worship his feet. The toes punishment was still the thing he made me do that I hated most and my stomach felt queasy at his words, but – heaven forgive me – I was so desperate to come that I began to move without hesitation, until him grabbing my hair stopped me.

'Actually Kate, before you do that, beg me to let you lick my toes.'

'What?' I snapped. I couldn't help myself.

'Beg me. You're going to beg me to lick and suck and worship my feet and if you do it well then I will let you. And when you put your mouth around my toes if you are a good girl I'll push a finger inside you. I wonder how wet I'll find you when I do.'

I whimpered. I knew the humiliating answer to that and both yearned for and dreaded the moment when he felt it for himself.

Thankful for the darkness in the room that meant I didn't have to look him in the eyes, I asked him if I could worship his feet. He pulled my hair back and demanded I speak up so Sarah could hear clearly.

With a voice filled with loathing and tears I just about managed a second go. 'Please, I am begging you to let me suck your toes.'

'Just to suck my toes?'

God I hated him. God he made me wet.

'No, to kiss them, to lick them, to clean them with my tongue. I want to worship your toes. All of your feet.' I was hoping I'd got most eventualities covered, but every word was laced with aggression and frustration so I thought I'd better moderate my tone a little: 'Please. Sir.'

He patted the side of my face, a gesture of tenderness which made everything else seem a little easier to bear, for a second, until he spoke again. 'You are a good slut. You may.'

Thank fuck. I crawled down and pushed my face into his toes, steeling myself for the first taste as I heard him give Sarah a running commentary. As I pulled his big toe into my mouth and began running my tongue up and down it, he explained to her how greedily I was taking it, and pushed his foot in further. He told her how he was making me clean him up properly by wiping his feet on my face and demanding I licked the undersoles. She was clearly quite horrified at the idea and, as he told her how he'd been wearing big walking boots and socks for most of the day and hadn't showered before bed, I heard her shriek in disgust and then giggle at my predicament – her words indistinct but the tone of her amusement carrying loudly across the room.

Silent tears dripped from my eyes as I did what he asked, unwilling to show him how far he'd pushed me but still desperate to continue. As he pushed one finger up inside my knickers I gasped, and he took the opportunity to push his foot further into my mouth.

As I focused on the feeling of his fingers between the folds of my dripping cunt I heard him say, 'She is such a filthy slut. She's dripping she's so wet. It's not going to take much to push her over the edge.' And then, after the mumbling sound of Sarah saying something at her end of the line he stopped and pulled his hand out. As I whimpered in frustration round his foot and he wiped his wet hand on my arse he said: 'That's a great idea,' and my blood chilled.

'Kate? You may stop worshipping my foot now.'

Normally those words would fill me with joy. As it was I was filled with terror. Would I get to come? Would I be able to stop myself from bursting into tears if I was going to be left frustrated? What was a good idea? If they were going to let me come what were they going to do with me that was worse than the foot thing? Would I want them to do anything? Would I rather go without? Could I rather go without? Almost hysterical thoughts ran through my mind of all the horrible things they could do to me, make me do. I knew, if there was anything utterly terrible I could refuse, end the game, except in that moment I had no intention of doing that, a hostage to my own desperate needs, which meant the possibilities terrified me. And in the end what they came up with between them was something that hadn't even crossed my – let's admit it – pretty twisted mind.

It was Sarah's idea, something that one day I will properly thank her for in person – preferably by watching her have to go through exactly the same thing. As Russell told me what I was to do I shut my eyes and pressed my lips together, shaking my head in silent rebellion, unwilling and unable to consider doing it. As the silence lengthened I realised this was it, that if I didn't do this I wasn't getting to come. For long seconds I tried to think of another way. Anything else I could. But slowly, grudgingly I accepted my fate.

And then I moved into position.

I knelt straddling one of his legs, looking through the darkness at him lying propped up slightly on the pillows with the phone to one ear, thinking if I could only just see him at least he would only vaguely be able to see me. I'd like to say that helped, but actually it didn't. I knelt there for a couple of seconds, unwilling to continue even while in my head I had surrendered to the knowledge that I would be doing so. That I was, right now, going to hump his leg like an animal to get my orgasm.

One of the things I find particularly interesting about the D/s dynamic is that it pushes you to do things that otherwise you might not do. Not because you don't want to – so often you really really do – but because it's stuff that intellectually while you think it's going to be hot / fun / interesting / unusual there's a small part of your mind that for whatever reason baulks at it – whether that's because you feel it's 'dirty', or it's too embarrassing or you're worried your arse'll look like a small country or whatever. I love that I can be pushed past the small part of my mind that feels that to experience these amazing new things is wrong. And no, that's not being pushed into doing something I don't want to do, coerced or whatever – my body betrays that it's something I'm into even if my eyes or words might for a time not make that obvious, even if I can't exactly explain why or how it's making me wet – but more about someone knowing how far I'd like to go and helping me find the courage to go for it.

Russell does that, often seemingly (and irritatingly) effortlessly. Mainly he tends to make it happen by striking a chord with my stubborn side where my response is to think 'no, I *am* going to do this, you can't come up with anything I don't feel comfortable doing' even while I feel hideously uncomfortable. Generally I enjoy that dichotomy, enjoy being pushed out of my comfort zone, doing things that make my stomach drop with nerves and make me blush with fury and embarrassment even as I get wet. But leg humping? Suddenly I was thinking fondly of his bloody feet. I hated it. Hated the idea of it. The indignity, the awkwardness of the angle I'd need to grovel at to actually do it, the fact I'd been fantasising about how he'd make me come for five fucking days and instead of it being any of the things I'd thought of, I'd have to do it myself. And not in a lovely way, not curled up with my hand between my legs, or with my favourite toy from the drawer, humping him like a bitch on heat. I felt rooted to the bed. I couldn't do this. I couldn't.

'Are you feeling embarrassed? Like you don't want to do this?' His voice had a sing-song mocking quality which was blatantly due to him playing to our telephonic audience. It made me feel murderous. OK, more murderous.

I cleared my throat and started to answer, my voice stuttering and unsure, but he interrupted me. 'I don't care. I've ordered you to hump my leg. We both know you're going to do it eventually one way or another because if you don't then you're not getting another chance to come before New Year, so if I were you I'd make it easier for yourself and start. Now.'

So. I humped him.

Fine, there's more to it than that. A lot more. And I'm not that much of a tease. But actually, honestly, even writing about it makes me feel prickly with embarrassment, a little sick with humiliation. And let's face it, I'm hardly shy about this stuff.

I hated it. Not in a "pretending to hate it but secretly quite liking it" way but in an "I actually hate it so much it is irritating and surprising to me that I might come doing this, bearing in mind how much it bothers me, how much it takes me out of the moment, how much it makes me want to tell Russell to go fuck himself" way. As I said, I get that only submitting to fun stuff isn't submission and I agree, which is why I didn't push Russell over and bugger off home to my comfy bed and full toy drawer. But humping his knee, trying to grind myself on it at the right angle that I could catch my clit and come and end the indignity even while he was deliberately shifting slightly to stop that happening and prolong my agony, all while (of course) he sat there telling Sarah how wet I was making his leg, how I was crying and yet my breathing was beginning to increase as I got closer to my orgasm, what a pathetic desperate horny slut I was... It made me furious. Flashbacks-for-days-afterwards-and-I-couldn't-think-clearly furious. It wasn't painful, not even that humiliating on paper. It sounds like such a little thing. I humped his leg. But it wasn't and I still can't get my head round why not, much less explain it. If I started writing about D/s in part because I enjoy the intellectual pursuit of trying to explain what I'm feeling and why the things that arouse me arouse me, then this is the thing that is so unexplainable to me that I may as well try and explain it in Flemish.

So I humped his leg, like an animal, while he gave Sarah a running commentary of how I was grinding myself against his knee, using the friction to provide my clit with the sensation I needed to come.

I ground myself against him, thinking how low I had sunk, how degraded and humiliated I had become in pursuit of my pleasure. Tears streamed down my face, trickling down my chin to cool my chest – flushed with embarrassment at the picture, thankful for the darkness which hid the worst of it. Practically speaking, it was an awkward position to get any kind of stimulation from. Russell was lying with his legs flat on the bed, and only by spreading mine widely around him and bending myself low to the bed could I even get close enough to his knee to push myself against him with the level of pressure I needed to get close to coming. I tried, oh how I tried, desperate to have this end, for me to have my orgasm and for this to be over.

Now you'd think that after five days of no orgasms, all that time I'd thought about sex, how desperate and aching and horny I was, that I would have come quickly. But, of course, the mind is a funny, twisted, and occasionally horrible thing. Knowing Sarah was listening to me doing this humiliating thing, hearing my moans and gasps of pleasure as – in spite of myself, my humiliation and my horror – I was wet and aroused and vociferously, shamefully taking pleasure from Russell's knee of all things, made me falter, as did hearing Russ tell her how he could hear the slurping sound of me sliding against his knee I had made him so wet. I tried blocking it all out, tried grinding harder, but I couldn't get the pressure I needed to bring myself off and end it.

'I can't –' I swallowed back some tears and some snot, cleared my throat and tried again. 'This angle isn't going to work. I'm not going to be able to come like this.'

'Well, what do you want me to do about that?' he sneered. 'You know what you have to do, and I'll be honest, I'm getting impatient now at having you grinding on me, making me whole leg wet. I'd hurry up if I were you.'

The thought of having gone through all this and still not getting to come made fear cramp my stomach.

'Your knee, if you could just raise your knee a little bit, that would make it easier. Please.'

I thought I saw his teeth flash in the darkness. 'Are you begging me to move my knee to make it is easier for you to hump it now?'

87

There was a pause. I had to moisten my lips with my tongue before I could speak and even then my voice was wavering and filled with tears. Normally I'd have prevaricated, tried to avoid this, but frankly I was broken, desperate, haunted. Every fibre of my being was desperate to come. 'Yes. Yes I'm begging you.'

'Good. Well beg me properly, louder, so Sarah can hear exactly how desperate you are, so desperate you're rubbing yourself against me like an animal on heat.'

My hands were clenched tightly, my fingernails digging into my palms as my voice filled the room. 'I am begging you. Please, Sir, lift your knee a little bit so I can grind against it–'

He interrupted me: 'No, 'hump it'.'

I sighed but didn't even pause: '–hump it until I come on your knee. Please.'

As he pushed his knee up, with force enough it bashed against my pubis in a way that zinged through me like a welcome electric shock, his voice was smug: 'There. That wasn't so difficult was it? Now make yourself come for me.'

The change in angle made all the difference. Suddenly the movement of my hips against the delicious friction of his knee was rubbing perfectly against my clit. I tried to block out as he told Sarah how suddenly I had started bucking like a madwoman, more desperate than ever, tried to ignore the sound of my arousal as I slid up and down against his knee, tried to block out everything but the pleasure beginning to thrum through my body, trying to overcome all the obstacles between me and the release I had been craving for the best part of a week.

I was crying in humiliation and horror by the time my orgasm neared although, inevitably, it didn't slow me down. As the shudders began running through me my sobs got louder. I spasmed around Russell's leg, like an animal, my high-pitched cries loud enough for Sarah to hear down the phone. After days of pent-up frustration my release was body-juddering and intense. Never in my life have I felt an orgasm like it, and for a second or two afterwards my world went dark as I lay there, my limbs trembling with the force of it. Once I came back to myself, I became aware of Russell wanking above me. I went to crawl up his body, but he stopped me with a tut.

'I don't think so. You need to clean your mess first.'

I knew what he meant and it should have filled me with fury but my head space was such that without demur I crawled over and began licking my juices clean off his knee, well actually most of his leg – I had managed to make him sticky from his mid-thigh down to his lower shins, much to my shame. I kept licking as he told Sarah what I was doing. I kept licking as he rubbed himself, aroused by and enjoying this final humiliation. I kept licking as he spunked on the side of my face and into my hair. Finally, as his cum dripped down my cheek, he held the phone closer to my ear and I heard Sarah orgasm.

Yes. The first time I heard Sarah on the phone she was coming. Even I will concede my world is at times an odd one. It was a bloody memorable Christmas holiday though.

Chapter Seven

OF COURSE IF LISTENING to someone you've never spoken to before orgasm on the phone is a slightly odd experience, then meeting her for a beer a few weeks later is, well, even more disconcerting really.

Russell had been chatting regularly on one of the online communities and when they organised a munch he was keen to go along and say hello to everyone. Once I realised that a munch was essentially a gaggle of people going out for drinks and possibly dinner and wasn't signing me up to an evening strapped naked to a St Andrews cross being flayed by random people as they walked past to go to the buffet table, I was happy to join him. Especially when I realised it meant I could meet Sarah, and thank her for the whole humping thing, in person.

So one Sunday afternoon we went to a pub in leafy North London, and had a beer and a lovely roast dinner – there's nothing better than pork with crackling and home-made Yorkshire puddings – with a couple of dozen interesting and kinky people.

The first thing of note was that, well, most people weren't really of note. Now I don't mean that it in a rude or disparaging way, but more that if I'd seen them walking down the street I would never have pegged them as being smutty types. They were all casually dressed (no gimp masks or PVC to be found), intelligent, articulate, warm people just having a chat and getting to know each other.

Being a people watcher, I enjoyed guessing where things would develop. Carol and Neil – a couple from up north who had moved down when Neil got a good job as a deputy head in a school just outside London – were chatting animatedly and with a fair amount of dirty-sounding laughter with Bev and Ian, who owned a business importing sustainable furniture from China. Meanwhile Ciara, who had been single for a while and had spent months merrily telling everyone actually she preferred it that way until she found someone special to play with, was fiddling with her glass and smiling widely while chatting to Jo in a way that made me hope she might have actually found what she'd been looking for. Russell meanwhile was moving from group to group, chatting comfortably to loads of different people in the way he does that I always find engaging and envy a little – despite being able to hold up my end of polite conversations in work situations I'm not naturally chatty and given half a chance would be sitting in the corner with a couple of people I know rather than, in the vernacular, working the room.

Not that I was given half a chance to be anything even remotely resembling a wallflower. Sarah made a beeline for us when she entered the beer garden, and when she came over, took my hand and pulled me up and into a hug my fingers tingled. Her touch was cool and firm. Her grip was stronger than I'd anticipated and she held my hand longer than expected as she looked into my eyes. Suddenly I was buzzing – and it wasn't from the glass of Shiraz I'd been nursing for most of the afternoon.

The spark surprised me. I'd had a bit of a bisexual

phase at university and had slept with a few women since, but it was rare for me to feel such an intense attraction to someone I'd just met. I could see why Russell was attracted to her. She was stunning. Elfin features, green eyes, a short haircut which showed off the nape of her neck.

I'm a sucker for the nape of the neck. There are other places you could stroke which will make me squirm faster and harder, but for my money the neck is an overlooked erogenous zone. I wanted to stroke her there and see if it made her squirm. I wanted to kiss my way down to her shoulders, pull open her shirt and work my way further down until I was in a position to find out whether her hair colour was natural.

As we sat making small talk I learned little things about her that made me like her more. She was intelligent and quick-witted and we had similar taste in everything from cheesy popcorn flicks to a shared loathing of Dan Brown. She had a dirty laugh and the way she licked her lips every time she took a sip from her vodka and Coke made me think very rude things indeed – and restrain the urge to forget our surroundings and lean over to run my own tongue over her mouth.

By the time we'd eaten lunch we were firm friends, although I still hadn't forgiven her for the humping, much to her amusement. Russell stopped mingling and came to sit with us in time for some dessert and a fair amount of smutty flirtation and mocking. The dynamic was fun, comfortable and – barring the teasing that saw me nicknamed Humpy for part of the afternoon and blushing accordingly – rather sexy.

Sarah was unconsciously, unfussily, attractive, with the kind of carefree doesn't-give-a-shit attitude that was both refreshing and made her beauty all the more natural and appealing. Whether she was winding a twisted tendril of her hair around a finger as she talked or gesticulating wildly while doing an impression of her boss everything she did was honest and raw and emotive – and, frankly, sexy as hell. And, as the wine flowed more freely, she told me exactly how things had felt from her end of the phone conversation, gnawing slightly on her full lower lip as she told me how hot I had sounded begging Russell to firstly let me kiss his feet and then let me come.

I flushed as the memories of what I had said, how desperate I had felt, flooded through my mind, and suddenly the atmosphere round our table shifted imperceptibly. I felt my nipples harden, but seeing Sarah's had done the same through her pale blouse made me feel slightly less disconcerted. We looked at each other, recognised our mirrored predicament, both moved to put our arms across our chests, and giggled, embarrassed co-conspirators. I shifted slightly in my seat, my hair falling in front of my face as I moved, hiding the worst of my blush, but she moved forward to tuck a strand behind my ear. She stroked my hair and I blushed harder, resisting the sudden urge to turn my head and kiss her fingers. Russell watched our exchange intently, but said nothing.

Of course, Russell not expressing an opinion on something is pretty much a sign of impending apocalypse and only lasts for a finite period of time. After we'd dropped Sarah off at the station and were in the car heading back to his house he was more relentless than Jeremy Paxman after a bag of Haribo.

'You seemed to get on really well. Did you like her?'

'Did you find her attractive?'

'Did her touching your face and stroking your hair like that make you wet?'

'Did you want to kiss her?'

By the time we'd got back to his house I was ready to burst.

'Yes! I liked her. She was sexy and lovely and fun. Happy? Now will you shut up?'

I know. It was an uncharacteristically pissy response. The thing is, I bet you're thinking it's because I was jealous of Russell turning his attention to someone else. In a way, that would make sense. But I wasn't jealous about Sarah potentially getting to play with my dom-with-benefits, actually I was a little grumpy about the idea of him getting to play with her. I liked her.

In the weeks that followed, Russell continued chatting to Sarah, and they met a couple of times. It gave me some pause for thought. Their relationship wasn't developing into a monogamous dating-type arrangement yet – the first giveaway being Russell happily tying me down with a plug in my arse, caning me and fucking me a couple of days after he told me they first slept together – but somehow the dynamic between us was changing a little and I began to think about the fact that there might come a time when we had to stop playing together. While I know lots of people who are happy with more casual relationships, polyamory and the like, I just didn't think that would be me, or Russell for that matter. Every time I submitted to him it felt more intense – with a small voice whispering that it might be the last time he clamped my nipples, or the last time he used his belt on me, the last time he fucked my arse. We talked about Sarah often – both in the bedroom when he would whisper filthy comments that made me wet about what it would be like if she was in the room with us, and outside it. I talked to her directly a fair bit too, but apart from a flirty evening where we went out for drinks it was all fairly innocent.

Until the bank holiday weekend.

We'd made plans to get together for a barbecue at Russell's house. The weather was gorgeous, and Sarah and I had both brought stuff to stay over so we could have a drink without worrying about having to get home.

The afternoon was lazy. Sarah and I lay in the garden, enjoying the warmth of the sun on our skin and trying for a bit of a tan, while Russell threw a frisbee for the dog, fired up the barbecue and pottered about, seemingly incapable of staying still. We ate a leisurely meal and then lingered at the table talking about nothing in particular, taking advantage of the good weather.

As the light changed and the shadows lengthened, the talk turned flirtier. Sarah told me she loved my breasts in the vest top I'd been wearing to tan my shoulders. I leant over to wipe some stray potato salad from her mouth. Meanwhile Russell sat, watching steadily, his gaze assessing in a way that normally meant only one thing.

In typical fashion he took the initiative, although I wondered if in part if that was because he'd had similar conversations with Sarah to the ones he'd had with me. In further typical fashion, he was characteristically blunt. Really blunt. In an "I wish I could make this sound more alluring than it was" sort of way.

'Shall we all go upstairs and fuck?'

Sarah and I looked at each other and burst out laughing. She pulled my hand into hers and smiling at me said, 'I think I'd quite like that.'

I rolled my eyes. 'Well with an offer like that, who could say no?' But inside I was giddy.

Russell sprang into action with all the energy of a natural planner – he'd definitely given this some thought.

Stacking up the plates to take indoors he told me to go upstairs and strip and wait for them on my hands and knees on the bed facing away from the door. While the idea of being the first one naked made me feel rather embarrassed, I knew that disobeying at this juncture would stall things before they started, as well as – let's face it – potentially storing up trouble for myself later on in the process.

I nodded and went upstairs to his bedroom.

I'm not a patient person. Kneeling there obediently waiting for the bedroom door to open, my stomach filled with butterflies and my nipples already erect at the prospect of what was to come, took all my self-control. There was no clock to look at, I wasn't wearing a watch, and it felt like ages. How long did it take to load a dishwasher anyway?

By the time I heard movement I was half convinced they had started downstairs without me and was pondering whether I could tiptoe downstairs quietly enough to not disturb them and see. Thankfully I didn't as then, finally, the door opened. It took all my self-control not to look round, but I knew I did so at my peril. Instead I stared intently at the pattern on the bedcover in front of me, while listening for any noise which might give a hint of what would happen.

The only thing I heard was … a quiet creaking?

As Sarah walked to stand beside me I realised why. She'd changed into a gorgeous leather corset, which she was wearing with knickers and stockings only. My throat felt dry. She was stunning and her elaborate outfit made me feel even more self-conscious in my nakedness.

Russell walked round to the other side of the bed, pausing to stand opposite her, leaving me in the middle, not sure where to look first, or even if I should be looking anywhere other than down at the fixed point on the coverlet of the bed. Finally, when it felt like the silence would never end, Russell broke it.

'Are you ready?'

I opened my mouth to reply, but before I could Sarah did. 'Yes.'

'Good girl. Just remember what we discussed.'

Before I could even begin to unravel what that meant, Russell was moving to the foot of the bed. Standing directly in front of me, he took my chin in his hand, pushing my face up to look into his eyes. 'You want to please me, don't you? Obey me?'

My usual feelings of wanting to please and yearning for a challenge to overcome were still there, but overshadowed by a fear in the pit of my stomach that actually I was about to be asked to do something more intense than I could imagine. My voice was quiet, betraying my confusion. 'Yes.'

He stroked my hair and for a second the affection of the movement soothed me. Until his words sank in. 'Good. Because right now I am going to sit down and leave you in Sarah's capable hands. She's always wanted to try her hand at being dominant but lacked the confidence to do so. I told her she could play with you. Try some things out. You should obey her as you would obey me. I'm watching.'

And with that he moved to sit on the comfy chair in the corner of the room which was normally covered with clothes but had, I now noticed, been cleared off for the occasion.

As Sarah moved towards me I felt a surge of fury and confusion. What the fuck was he playing at? Did she really think I'd submit to her? And since when did she want to dominate anyone anyway? It would seem I didn't know Sarah as well as I'd thought.

She crouched down a little to meet my eyeline. 'You're going to hump my leg tonight, Kate,' she told me.

Mentally I rolled my eyes. It would seem Sarah didn't know me as well as she thought either. My tone was mocking. 'You think so? That's sweet. Wrong, but very sweet.'

There is a whole subculture of submissive women that focus on being contrary, disobedient, brattish. Women who enjoy acting out of line, so they can be pulled back into it, punished into submission. Now don't get me wrong, I'm as fond of being overpowered by someone stronger than me as the next woman, but generally where I can obey I will do. There are things I baulk at and will do grudgingly and with embarrassment, but for the most part my submission is more about doing something to please the person I am playing with. I'm not, generally, a brat.

But looking up at Sarah, even dressed in that gorgeous corset which did such amazing things to her body, something clicked in my mind. I can be pretty stubborn at the best of times, but this was different, stronger than that. I was adamant. I was not going to submit to her just because Russell said I should.

Does that make me a bad sub? A disobedient one? Probably, yes. But let's face it, it's not as if through the entire process I'd been the Stepford Sub and this was suddenly a break away from the norm. In my mind my submission is a gift, something to be earned, and while I gave it freely to Russell, the idea of giving it to Sarah, even at his behest, brought me up short.

I stared back at her steadily, not exactly glaring, but not looking in any way submissive. It was a look I knew I would never get away with in front of Russell in a million years, but frankly I didn't give a toss.

Neither of us spoke. Out of the corner of my eye I could see Russell smiling slightly. I was fearful he would intervene, and not entirely sure how I would respond if he pushed this whole "submitting to her is submitting to him" line. But he seemed amused more than anything else and keen to see how things would play out.

Slowly, deliberately, Sarah moved closer. And then she slapped my face. Hard. It stung and I felt myself going red – not just where she'd struck me but across my entire face and neck – in fury and embarrassment at the slight. For a split second I thought about slapping her back, but before the germ of the thought could flourish she'd grabbed a handful of my hair and yanked me towards her to kiss me.

I had spent a long time wondering what kissing Sarah would be like, but I had never expected it to be like this. She tasted of mint and smelled of flowers, but while her lips were as soft as I had fantasised they would be, her hand in my hair and the way she kissed me made me whimper a little as she took control of the kiss, and of me. Her tongue pushed inside me, her teeth nipped at my mouth, her hand pulled my hair, bending me to her will until I was compliant underneath her.

She pulled away and the spell was broken. I knew I was gaping at her a little, my mouth swollen from her kisses, and her teeth. As she moved her hand back to my face it took all my self-control not to flinch, betraying my nerves. But I had nothing to fear, instead of slapping me again, she stroked my face gently.

'We'll see, shall we?'

In all honestly, at that moment I had no recollection at all what she was talking about. Instead my mind was reeling at this gorgeous woman who I was beginning to think I might have underestimated.

As she stroked my hair her voice had taken on a different timbre too. It wasn't a dom voice – or I suppose technically a domme voice – in Russell's style, but she was assured and unwavering. She had no doubts that whatever she was going to do would make me submit, and that made me nervous. What the fuck had the two of them been discussing over the same weeks Russell was asking me whether thoughts of her breasts made me wet?

'We've been talking about you, Kate. About how stubborn you can be. How disobedient.'

I bloody knew it.

'The thing is, Kate, I don't intend to have you disobey me. I think you want to obey me, deep down. And I'm going to make sure that you do.'

I closed my eyes for a few seconds so she didn't see me rolling them.

'We talked about what to do when you don't obey.'

Eyes opened now, I kept looking ahead, trying to zone out a little. I wasn't expecting her to be able to push my emotional buttons quite this easily, and had no intention of rising to her bait.

'So tell me. What does Russell do when you do things you're not supposed to?'

In spite of myself I began to feel myself blush. I knew what I was supposed to say and I was a little concerned now at the prospect of disobeying her. But I hated admitting this stuff aloud at the best of times. Saying it to her then, like that? The dual submission – not just to her but to the part of me that wanted this, needed this, gets turned on by the humiliation of it – stuck in my throat.

As I tried to gather my thoughts she slapped me again.

In my peripheral vision I saw Russell move forward to better watch my reaction.

'Answer me. What happens?'

I cleared my throat, wondering why this felt so humiliating, trying hard to soften my tone in a way that didn't betray the extent to which it does.

'He punishes me.'

Her hand twisted in my hair, a tug of warning. 'I didn't hear you.' Fuck, Russell had told her all his best moves, this woman was dangerous. Part of me loathed her and the other part of me was getting more aroused by the minute.

Louder: 'He punishes me.'

'Better. How does he punish you?'

My temper was rising – she knew how he punished me because he'd told her, no doubt gloating about the things he could get me to do, do to me. She knew, he knew and I knew and yet she was making me say it out loud because she knew it makes me embarrassed. I was angry and I was wet and that I could feel myself getting wetter as I knelt on the bed in front of them only made me more angry.

I tried to hide the annoyance but I could hear the sharpness in my voice. 'It depends. Whip. Belt. Cane. Crop. Hand. Whatever he wants.'

As she moved away from me and the link between us was broken for a moment I expelled the breath I hadn't even realised I was holding. For a second the relief was palpable, until she returned, holding something that made my stomach fall.

As she tapped me gently on the shoulder with the cane I began trembling uncontrollably. Surely he wasn't going to let her …?

'I've always wondered what it feels like to cane someone.'

Shit.

After the first six hits Russell took pity on me and moved closer to coach her. I'd have been grateful, but I was already weeping and frankly not sure he could do much to help. My mind was reeling at the agony she was inflicting, and I was trying to work out whether she'd either never been on the receiving end of the cane before or had been but hated it so much she wanted to share the misery.

The strikes kept going as Russ coached on the best way to hit me, when to flick from the wrist, when to use the full arm. The angle to take. How to mix between hitting places you've hit before and new places so you can watch the reaction to the different kinds of pain. When to hold back. When to push harder.

The pauses meant it was difficult to process the pain as there was no rhythm to it, no way of riding the peaks and troughs. Instead I retreated into it, only half aware of their discussion about the welts on my arse and how long they would take to go down as I listened intently for the swish of the cane through the air, trying to and prepare myself for the next wave of agony.

I don't know how long it went on but finally there was respite – four hands running over the marks, her fingernails tracing the lines marking the hot welts, he brutally squeezing the most punished part until I whimpered. Then, for the most fleeting moment, so gently that I wondered whether I was imagining it, a finger ran up my slit. I moaned in frustration as it moved away.

Her voice was filled with a quiet wonder. 'This is making her wet.'

She sighed in pleasure behind me and Russell chuckled. 'It's making you wet too.' His voice was pleased. She laughed and I feel a pang of jealousy.

Russell moved to me, running his finger briefly along the ridge between my top lip and my nose, before turning away. My frustration at this briefest of touches burned into an aroused fury a second later when her scent filled my nostrils. Listening to the sound of them kissing, touching, fucking even, inches away from me, knowing the wetness drying on my face was her juice, was erotic torture. But I didn't dare sneak a glance. I waited, docile, for them to turn their attentions back to me.

I can't tell you exactly when my mindset changed. It snuck up on me. One minute I was furious and embarrassed and a bit concerned at submitting to Sarah, and the next I was completely in the moment and none of that mattered any more.

After she'd finished with the cane, and Russell had finished with her – for then at least – she moved back into my field of vision and picked up the accursed paddle. As my inner monologue wondered for the thousandth time why the fuck I'd thought buying it was a good idea, she stared at the lettering cut into it and smiled.

'So this is the famous slut paddle.'

I looked up to answer as Russell replied. This keeping silent thing was not a natural state for me.

'This is the one. She hates it. Always concerned I'm going to mark her with it and she's going to end up caught out at the gym.'

Sarah smiled and I felt a little cramp of fear in my stomach. Had I not noticed the slightly sadistic curve of her lips before? Or had I inspired this? It made me wet and fearful at the same time, even as I knelt there, my arse in the air, waiting for what happened next.

'So it does work then? You can end up effectively branding her with 'slut'?'

Russell laughed. 'Well I can. Just about. It takes a lot

of effort and some big swings though. In a lot of ways it's even more precise than the cane. It only works if you hit her in the right spot, really really hard.'

As she moved behind me, for a split second, I hated him. And then all thoughts except enduring this faded from my mind.

Well you had to give her marks for trying. She hit me really hard, many times. I couldn't tell you how many, as all I was doing was trying to withstand them, to minimise my sobs and contain the worst of my shaking as the loud cracks rained down on my already burning arse. I don't know how effective I was at either if I'm honest.

There was no rhythm to her movements as, when she connected with a crack which she thought had made the mark, she stopped to check her handiwork. I would kneel there, hoping to hell that actually she *had* marked me, just because then at least she would stop. But then she would pick up the paddle and continue and the agony would start again. Suddenly any mental debate about whether I should or could or would submit to her was academic. Somehow, with that punishment, in that room, suddenly I was hers. It didn't occur to me to disobey her, although I wished she'd get the mark she wanted so she would stop hitting me.

After a while – a long while – she seemed to get bored trying. She dropped the paddle on the bed and, over my head, told Russell she'd be back in a moment.

As she left the room he moved closer and crouched down level to my face. As he brushed tears from my cheeks with his thumbs his voice was soothing.

'How are you doing? Are you OK? Are you enjoying this?'

I nodded, pressing my lips together to stop them

104

trembling, unable to even begin explaining in words exactly how I felt, knowing I might be able to after the event but that right now they were simply beyond me.

He smiled at me. 'Good. Because seeing you submit to her for me is so fucking hot. I love that you'll do anything for her because I tell you to.'

The usual running narrator of submission was there, protesting that actually I wouldn't do "anything" but it was fogged out, pushed away by the sensations, the myriad of tides of pain and the ebbing warmth of the pleasure between my legs. As the door reopened he leaned forward and kissed me, briefly and brutally, and then moved away.

The action surprised me, as did the tenderness of his mouth on mine. But in that moment, that kiss was a reminder of his dominance and it warmed me. Reassured me. Which was particularly good as suddenly he and Sarah were behind me, as she said: 'I didn't think it could happen, but I got bored of hitting her. Well actually, I'm not bored, my arm got tired.'

Russell laughed at the audible pout in her voice. I saw the humour, but didn't even smile, as I had to know what was coming next.

'I had another idea.'

Shit. This would be what was coming next.

There was a tickling feeling on my arse. After all the punishment I had taken that evening it should have felt like a welcome change, but actually it was just a different kind of pain, making my legs wobble, as it traced across the lines of the cane, the red fire of the paddling. It wasn't hard, but it was focused, like she was tracing her finger along my flesh.

Except I soon realised that it wasn't her finger.

Russell's murmur of appreciation was the first giveaway.

'I like that. Give me a go.'

More pressure, this time on the other arse cheek. A giggle from Sarah. I tried to turn my head subtly to catch even the briefest glimpse of what they were doing, but my movement caught Russell's attention and a twist of my nipple made it clear he wasn't allowing any such thing.

He tutted, and then said: 'It would appear Kate wants to see what we're doing. Should we show her?'

Sarah giggled again. 'I think we should turn her over and then she can see.'

Between them they manoeuvred me onto my back on the bed, Sarah making a little "awwww" of sympathy at my gasp of pain as I first landed on my arse.

She leaned forward to brush some hair out of my eyes, and I was reminded for a second of the smiling girl drinking wine and blushing sitting in a beer garden.

'I decided that rather than making my arm any more tired than it already was, I would write on you. The effect's the same and it's much simpler, don't you think?'

And then the girl from the beer garden was gone.

By the time they were finished my body was covered in insults, all in a rich, deep red lipstick. My arse marked me slut, obviously, but elsewhere I was whore, fuckhole, bitch, slave. And once they had finished writing on me they mauled me with their hands, amusing themselves by trying to make the lipstick smudge – "well all true sluts have smudged lipstick" – their touch making me writhe in pleasure, in spite of myself.

After a little while though, Sarah tired of the game, urging me forward so she could paint my mouth with the sticky, blood-red lipstick. As Russell stood beside her, I felt a pang at what a stunning couple they made – still dressed, pristine, sexy. I in comparison was a dishevelled mess – naked, covered in lipstick insults and marks from my punishment and with sticky thighs and a glistening cunt. The heavily painted red staining my mouth just finished it off.

As they kissed in front of me, Sarah urged me forward.

'On to your knees, I want you to show us how much of your master you can take in your mouth. I shall be checking his cock for how high the mark of your slutty lipstick comes, and if it isn't far enough I'm sure I can force myself to punish you a little more.'

On an ordinary day my inner monologue would have been screaming at the idea of Russell being my master, but I didn't give a toss. I moved from the bed eagerly, the pain of my arse ignored in my haste to sink to my knees in front of them both. I unzipped his trousers, pulling his cock out and putting my mouth around him, enjoying the taste of him, feeling him grow as I angled my head to suck him deeper. I felt Sarah move around me and suddenly I could hear the two of them kissing above me, as I kept sucking Russell's cock. Sarah's hand slid to my head and she stroked my hair. It was one of the most arousing things I have ever experienced. Well at least until they started fucking and I crawled up between them to fasten my mouth round Sarah's clit.

By the time Russell had come once and Sarah twice I was squirming with a desperate need to orgasm myself. All three of us were lying on the bed, Sarah gently stroking my arm while I pressed a kiss to her stomach.

'Would you like to come, Kate?'

I opened an eye suspiciously. I knew where this was going, and what was really awful was by this point I had no compunction about it, I knew I would hump her leg if I had to.

'Yes please.'

Her smile was beautiful and her mouth curved when she leant down to kiss me softly. 'Come on, Kate, you can do better than that. I've heard you beg before remember. I know how well you do it.'

I flushed, as both Russell and Sarah turned to look at me. Staring past them a little, stammeringly I managed to ask them, both – I wasn't risking a breach of etiquette at this point in proceedings – if they would please allow me to come.

Sarah tutted. 'Are you begging, Kate?'

I sighed. 'Yes, Sarah, I'm begging you. Please let me come.'

Sarah laughed at me. 'I will, if you kiss my arse.'

I'm fairly sure my eyes widened in comedy fashion. 'What?'

'Kiss my arse. And then, actually, I think I'd like to feel your tongue running up between my arse cheeks, lapping at my hole. If you do that, I'll let you come.'

I was agog. This was something I knew Russell wasn't into, would never ask me to do. I'd never worried about doing it, it just wasn't an option.

My body ached I was so desperate to come. But her arse?

Suddenly, Russell's voice was loud in my ear. 'I told you, she won't do it. Get her to hump your leg instead.'

I felt a twinge of fury, feeling like a piece of meat, something to discuss between themselves. Then Sarah moved closer, kissing me softly on the lips, looking intently at my face.

'Kate, I could make you hump my leg. You know if I slapped you or picked up that cane again you'd be weeping and begging me to do whatever I wanted very quickly. Between us Russell and I could hold you down, I could sit my arse on your face, I could force you. But I don't want to force you. I want you to submit to me willingly. I want you to crawl up here and worship my arse, to do something you've never done before and something I've never had anyone do to me before. And while you do it Russ will make you come. I don't want to punish you, but I do want your obedience. Yes, you've been obeying me because Russell gave you to me –' I wasn't sure this was entirely true but didn't want to interrupt her flow '–but I want you to do this for me. Just me. Now.'

The room was silent and still for a few seconds. I didn't move, but I knew exactly what I was going to do, that I was going to obey her.

I crawled gently up her body and pressed a kiss to her lovely smooth arse. And then as Russell pushed his fingers deeply inside me I began licking and kissing her in perhaps the most intimate way possible. It was a humiliation I had never considered, but in that room in that moment, she had convinced me. I submitted for her, not Russell, to please her, and did so eagerly. And as my tongue pushed into her arse she moaned in pleasure, reaching back to stroke my hair. And then I came, gasping and whimpering into her arse as the release juddered through me.

Once my mindblowing orgasm had dissipated a little, a smiling Sarah explained the bet that she and Russell had made. Russ was adamant that she would not have been able to get me to rim her and had told her that if she did she would get to fuck me with her newly acquired strap on. If she didn't, then she would be severely punished, ending her turn as top. As we continued long into the night, a tangle of limbs and combinations and some of the sexiest experiences I've ever had, I was very thankful indeed at being inspired to submission.

Although I did still owe Sarah some revenge for the whole leg-humping thing.

Chapter Eight

CONSIDERING ALL THE PLAY with Russell, and getting to meet and submit to Sarah, you'd think I'd have been happy with my lot in life. But Russell starting to get to know Sarah had made me realise that while I loved the dynamic between us and the fun we had, actually I was looking for something more. We were never going to date, I had come to that conclusion long ago, and the more I thought about it the more I realised I was after the whole bundle – someone who could be my partner and lover but with a dominant dimension that meant I was having as much fun fucking him as curling up on the sofa watching a film afterwards.

When I met Josh I thought he could be that person. Although actually he almost didn't become my dom at all.

I met him after he sent me a message through a kink site. After a few months of finding no wheat whatsoever in amongst the chaff of the semi-literate, the arsey, the downright rude, I had stopped replying to messages. I was bored with the cut and pasted emails, the typo-laden orders for me to "submit bitch, to ur Master" from men I had never spoken to before and yet seemed to think that as a sub I was going to subjugate myself like some kind of doormat automaton to everyone with a vaguely dominant tendency who appeared in front of me.

So all in all I was off replying to messages.

When I read the note he sent me something stopped me from deleting it with the half dozen others in my inbox that morning, but I absolutely was not going to reply. And the first day I didn't. But the next time I logged in I found myself rereading his message and tapping out a brief few lines of response. He was articulate, funny, and referred to the *West Wing*, which is a good barometer of character as far as I'm concerned. We started off just chatting about the world, the kind of small talk you'd make with someone you'd meet in a bar. And over a few weeks we chatted more and more, slowly finding out more about each other. Not just our kinks, although in spite of my best intentions I found myself wondering what it would be like to submit to him as he gave little hints as to things he had done previously, but also snapshots of our day-to-day lives and the things we had in common.

But I was still a bit dubious about him. In fact the sheer length of the list of things that I liked about him made me suspicious that he couldn't be that amazing at all. Self-preservation? Possibly. But also realism, as by this point I had spoken to lots of people who, if they hadn't lied about themselves outright online, could charitably at least have been said to have misrepresented themselves.

So I wasn't going to give him my instant messenger details. I wasn't going to submit to him on webcam. I wasn't going to give him my mobile phone number and start texting him. A few weeks later, once I had found myself at odd moments of the day thinking of the glint in his eye before he suggested something smutty, the way his lips curved when he smiled and pondering exactly what it would be like to suck his cock, I wasn't going to agree to meet him for dinner – nothing more to start with – in a gorgeous restaurant in Central London.

And I certainly wasn't going to be going home from

said dinner without any knickers, having taken them off and given them to him as per his order shortly before dessert.

Best laid plans and all that.

I know the knickers thing makes me sound like an utter slut. And I really didn't anticipate it. In fact I'd deliberately worn comfy non-date undies, so adamant was I that he wasn't going to see them the first time we met. And for most of the evening it didn't seem like it would be an issue.

I arrived late – a crisis at work from a late-developing story conspiring with train trauma – to find him sitting at the bar. He stood formally to greet me and first impressions were, well, great actually. I knew what he looked like from our sessions on webcam, but in the flesh I could see all those things that even the most megapixelled camera just can't show. He was much taller than I'd expected, his eyes shone with intelligence and good humour and I instantly felt comfortable with him. Which is probably just as well seeing everything that happened afterwards.

He was understanding about my tardiness, brushing aside my stammered apologies as we were shown to our table and seated. Over the next few hours we ate a leisurely meal, dragging it out in a way that if it had been anything other than a grim January Monday would have seen the waiting staff dropping hints that we should get the bill or adjourn back to the bar.

We talked about films, the media, argued about TV. It was fun, mentally challenging and punctuated with laughter. From the outside it would have looked like a vanilla date. Certainly someone passing our table might have noticed my face reddening at times, flushed as if I'd had a little too much wine. But they had no way of knowing that I was only drinking sparkling water and instead was squirming because Josh was discussing the 100 strikes with a drumstick I had accrued in punishments over the few months we had been chatting for various misdemeanours and how he was looking forward to seeing me bent over, counting and thanking him for every stroke, some time very soon.

At one point he invited me to come back to his place that evening, and while I demurred – even his charms could not circumvent basic common sense and the need for safety – there was part of me yearning to take him up on his offer. But as dinner progressed and my resolution wavered in spite of myself, he turned the tables again, changing his mind before I could change mine and declaring we should enjoy the anticipation. But anticipation only goes so far and we'd made plans to meet again before we'd even finished our supper. Forty-eight whole hours later. For what it's worth as we talked about it, it felt like eons away.

That was when the world beneath my feet shifted slightly. Having settled on a mutually convenient time for this second meeting, he leaned back in his chair, dabbed at his mouth with his napkin, set it down neatly on the table and told me I should give him a present before I left that evening. The atmosphere had shifted imperceptibly, his smile still as charming and as warm, just now with something else lurking beneath the surface. I pressed my hands together to hide the slight tremble in them and feigned insouciance as I asked what exactly he had in mind.

That's when he said: 'Your knickers.'

It took every ounce of effort to not flinch at all. Pride? Probably. A stubborn need to prove I wouldn't be fazed by any challenge he set me? Definitely. He waited silently for my response. I shifted in my seat.

With what I thought was a remarkably calm voice under the circumstances I inquired as to how this would work. As this was a from-work date and I'm hardly the girliest girl at the best of times I was wearing trousers. Would I be permitted to go to the bathroom to remove my knickers and then give them to him later?

He watched me intently as we discussed it, his smile getting wider until he was practically laughing at me outright. Foolhardy perhaps, and certainly not suitably subtly, but I couldn't stop myself from asking exactly what he found so funny.

He gestured at me. 'You're delightful. Your chin is up and your voice is casual. But your body betrays you.'

In spite of myself I felt my chin rising even further as I replied, trying for a calmness of tone that felt just a fingertip out of reach – although I hoped he didn't know me well enough to be able to pick up on that too.

'I don't know what you mean.'

He touched me, skin against skin, for the first time, and it felt like an electric shock surging through my body. His finger brushed the top of my hand as he spoke, stroking me in a way that felt oddly hypnotic, making my pulse race and my breathing get shallower as I tried to focus on what he was saying. In the tiny part of my brain that wasn't thinking about how surreal it was to be discussing the practicalities of giving my knickers to a man I'd just met for the first time three hours before, I wondered what pleasure – and pain – he could wring from my body, when with one finger he was already driving me to a kind of distraction.

'You're focusing hard on controlling your voice, your words. But your cheeks are flushed, and look at your hand –' he tapped gently on the top of it '– suddenly

115

clutching at the edge of the table for support.' I blinked and looked down to see my fingers gripping the dark wood, feeling like my hand belonged to someone else, seeing myself as he saw me, knowing he was right and blushing even harder. So much for remaining in control. Bugger. I unfurled my fingers and left my hand resting gently on the table, aiming for a casualness we both knew I wasn't feeling. I swallowed hard, fighting to regain a sense of equilibrium.

'I really don't know what you mean.'

He smiled again, almost indulgently, the way you would at an entertaining and yet naive child. 'I think you do. Perhaps you don't. But soon you will.'

And then he patted my hand one last time. 'Shall we get the bill?'

I came back from the toilet to find he had paid the bill and retrieved my coat, and was standing by the door looking out into the night. I walked the full length of the restaurant to join him, the seam of my trousers pressing against my slit with every step, a delicious friction exacerbated by my increasing wetness in the light of this slightly surreal turn.

As he helped me into my coat, he pressed a seemingly solicitous hand to the small of my back under my jacket to usher me out of the restaurant. Only I knew that he was actually sliding a finger under my waistband to see whether I'd obeyed his order. His murmur of pleasure when he realised I had thrilled me.

He walked me to the tube where we were to go our separate ways. As I stepped onto the down escalator he moved in behind me, his body pressing against mine, his breath tickling my neck as he whispered into my ear, filthy things that made me wetter. I bit my lip to stifle a moan as he told me what a slut I was and how I had pleased him with my obedience, and outlined the plans he had for me in a few days time.

As we walked towards the ticket barrier he grabbed my wrist, pulling me against a pillar to one side of the gate. Pressing me into the wall with his body, he anchored one hand in my hair and kissed me deeply, pillaging my mouth. His other hand was still around my wrist, pulling my hand down to feel his erection under his jacket. I felt shy, embarrassed – long past the age of snogging and copping a feel in public this way – but couldn't resist running my hand along the thickness of his cock, feeling him grow through his trousers.

He ended the kiss and we moved apart. He was looking at me expectantly, but for the life of me I couldn't work out what he wanted me to say. I wasn't actually sure I could form words. Eventually he smiled and held out his hand.

'I believe you have something for me.'

I closed my eyes for a second to try and mask my embarrassment at having momentarily forgotten all about it, having become so caught up in the kisses, before fumbling in my pocket to pull out my neatly folded pants. Of course I'd folded them, balling them up just seemed so uncouth somehow. I passed my knickers to him, focusing completely on ensuring my hand didn't shake, dreading he was going to unfurl them, sniff them, goodness knows what. He smiled, thanked me and put them in his pocket. I let out the trembling breath I hadn't realised I was holding, and as I did so he brushed one last kiss across my now swollen lips and leant to whisper in my ear.

'I am going to make you feel so fucking small when I see you on Wednesday. I can't wait.'

The words – particularly incongruous coming from the

lips of someone as well-spoken and impeccably polite –
were shocking and yet thrilled me to my core. I walked
away feeling like the entire evening had been magical and
yet unreal, my fingers brushing my still-wet mouth,
horny, amazed and terrified in about equal measure.

Suffice to say I was very thankful indeed I had replied
to his first message.

I have a terrible sense of direction. Awful. If there is one
characteristic about myself that I dislike above all others
it is the fact I am incapable of finding my way anywhere.
It makes me feel out of control, powerless, and not in a
good way. I've been known to get lost in people's houses.

Josh lived over the other side of the city to me. I
decided that driving was a sensible course of action as it
meant I could leave as early or as late as I wanted without
having to rely on public transport. Of course my crappy
navigation skills made for a stressful drive over, even
before I discovered his road was apparently the only one
I'd ever seen without a sign showing its name. Plus most
of my mind was focused on exactly what would happen
when I got there. I trusted him in the sense that I knew
enough of him that my nutter radar wasn't sounding, but I
knew playing with him would be intense – both because it
was the first time we were doing so and because he
seemed to have an innate ability to keep me on the back
foot. I had also had a serious case of the butterflies and
had done since I'd had a text from him a few hours
earlier:

*I am having concentration issues today. Keep thinking
about exactly what to do with you. x*

It pretty much scuppered the productivity of my
afternoon too as, with the best will in the world, cutting
down Women's Institute meeting reports for the village

news page is never going to hold the attention when your mind's pondering smut. I found myself unable to stop thinking about what he might be thinking about. I knew I had the punishment to come, although I wasn't especially bothered about it – while his use of a drumstick was apt because we'd been arguing about a video game which utilised the same, I was unconvinced he'd be able to use it to do any damage just because it was so unbendy. So apart from a hundred taps on the arse (I'd feign pain, didn't want to undermine his dom mojo) what else would he do? What would he have me do? Would he let me suck his cock? Would he fuck me? Remembering his final words to me as we parted at the tube, how small would he make me feel? How small could he make me feel anyway? What did that even mean?

An attempt at reasserting some semblance of control didn't end especially well. When I sent him a text asking if I could bring anything with me, I was thinking a bottle of wine or dessert. But his response was unequivocal and made my cunt clench as I sat at my desk.

Nipple clamps. x

Oh my. Suffice to say the WI didn't get anywhere near the level of professional attention they should have done that afternoon.

Finally I arrived at what I was fairly sure must be his road, parked my car and walked over to what I was hoping was his door. I rang the doorbell and as he came down to greet me, barefoot and smiling, I found myself smiling back in spite of my nerves. We walked up the stairs to his flat, although my distractedness was such that I managed to walk halfway up his stairs before he turned to look at me and said, 'Kate? You need to close my front door.'

Oooops. I blushed, went back down the stairs and

closed it, before walking back up trying to look as if nothing had happened. Smooth. I know, I impress myself with my ability to hold it together in challenging social situations.

We got into the flat and he directed me to the living room so I could put my handbag down. I walked in, and turned around, taking the opportunity to scope out the shelves and clutter for more clues about the kind of man he was – I know this makes me sound like a stalker, I maintain it's my journalistic tendencies, although some people might argue that's the same thing. Then he cleared his throat.

'Close the door please, Kate.'

I was halfway across the room to obey before I realised I'd moved instinctively. I shut the door gently and turned round, to find him right behind me, invading my personal space. His hands entwined into my hair as he bent his head towards mine for a kiss. I closed my eyes, enjoying the moment, how he towered over me, held me in place as his tongue invaded my mouth. He was the tallest man I had kissed, and – not being short myself – it was a novelty to feel dwarfed by his size. I felt he could either protect or overpower me easily depending on his intent.

As he broke away and moved his mouth towards my ear, I felt very strongly that his intent in this particular instance was the latter.

His voice was as well-spoken as ever as he hissed into my ear. 'You're a slut. We both know it. You've spent weeks thinking about what it would be like to suck my cock and now you're going to find out. I'm going to let you taste my spunk before dinner. I want to fuck your mouth. Get down on your knees. Now.'

He moved back slightly so he could watch my reaction. The room was silent. Still. We looked at each other for long seconds. He raised an eyebrow in a way that felt like he was both mocking and challenging me, that made the argumentative part of me chafe and long to butt heads with him, even while I found it – him – sexy. Since the dinner two nights ago this had been an inevitability. I wanted to submit to him, had been dreaming of it. I found him attractive, knew he would dominate me in a way that would provide great pleasure for both of us. But as he stared down at me, so secure in the fact that I was going to sink to my knees, part of me felt furious. I hadn't even taken my fucking coat off yet.

I wanted to tell him to knob off, was fairly sure that my mutinous glare was probably saying just that. But as I looked into his eyes I knew the only way all the amazing things I had spent weeks pondering would happen was if I obeyed him now. Right now. It was time to put up or shut up.

I put up. Or 'put out' perhaps is more apt.

I sighed slightly and sank to my knees, thrilled and yet irritated by the smirk of satisfaction on his face as he watched me settle myself at his feet.

He stroked my hair. 'Good girl.'

Being called a girl is one of the things that makes me bristle more than any other – along with being described as "feisty". But while part of me bridled at the patronising nature of the endearment, another part revelled in his praise, keen to show him exactly how good I could be. I leaned forward, opened his fly and gently pulled his cock out. I took my time, running my tongue up and down his shaft, before sucking it fully into my mouth. As I did so though he grabbed the back of my head and began pushing himself into me, leaving me gasping around him. We were battling for control of the rhythm. I struggled to take him, and he took his pleasure at his own pace. As I gasped around his cock he pulled out, a moment of relief.

As my breathing slowed he rubbed his cock, sticky with my saliva and his precum across my cheek, anointing my face with our mixed juices. Writing it down it seems like such a little thing, but my first instinct was pure fury. Feeling him rub the stickiness over my face made me flush with anger. I clenched my hands at my sides, fought to control the loud voice in my head screaming out to rebel, to pull away. No one had ever treated me that way before and it felt so degrading that it took all my effort not to react, instead to let him continue. Despite the part of me that enjoyed it, the greater part of me was furious.

The strength of my reaction threw me for a minute. Fighting to control myself, I closed my eyes against the view to block it out, mask my response to it, taking deep breaths to do everything I could to continue the submission in spite of myself. With my eyes shut the slap was a surprise. It didn't hurt exactly, although it felt like enough of a blow that I opened my eyes to see what he had done – just in time to see close up as he hit me in the face for a second time with his cock. I moaned in humiliation, as he continued his assault, his hand in my hair holding me in place as he used me, alternately slapping me and rubbing his cock across my face. I was disgusted, debased, and yet – inevitably – oh so wet. I shifted slightly on my knees to try and subtly remove the sticky gusset of my knickers away from my slit.

He slapped me once more with his cock, before grabbing a clump of my hair and forcing his cock back into my mouth. I opened as wide as possible to accommodate him, running my tongue up his cock as fast as he fucked my face. Then – so suddenly that I almost choked when the first spurt hit the back of my throat – he came in my mouth. As I swallowed him down and began licking him clean he pulled away from me, putting his cock back in his boxers and doing up his trousers.

I knelt there at his feet, unsure what was to happen now, my cunt wet, my nipples hard in my bra, and the taste of his spunk in my throat. He stroked my hair for a second before reaching down to take my arm and solicitously help me to my feet.

'Let me take your coat. And now let's just go and cook some dinner and relax for a little while.'

Feeling not unlike Alice having fallen down a sexy and yet mind-boggling rabbit hole, I took my coat off and followed him into the kitchen. I had been in his house for about ten minutes.

I love home cooking. Seriously. A great home-cooked dinner means more to me than the swishest restaurant. Living alone means I tend to not bother for the most part, living on stir-fry, soup and cereal. Every so often I'll go the other way and make something elaborate, although what usually happens is I get halfway through the process and am bored by the chopping, stuffing and basting and then revert back to soup for another three months.

So being around anyone who can cook is always a welcome novelty. As I sat on a stool in his kitchen with a glass of wine, Josh pottered around, chopping vegetables and crushing garlic for a mushroom risotto. We chatted about work and TV, and generally it was comfortable and relaxed and felt a million miles away from what had just happened in his bedroom. Of course the change of gear left me completely on the back foot. And obviously, being me, I was doing everything I could to show that I wasn't in any way bothered at all. In fact if it wasn't for the fact my body was crying out to come, I'd have thought I'd imagined it all.

As it was, dinner was lovely, the company was good, as was the conversation. We watched a bit of telly as we ate, and through it all at least three-quarters of my conscious thought was about sex. Frankly if the risotto hadn't tasted amazing it would probably have been more. At one point I had to make a deliberate effort to stop my hand shaking around my glass such was the level to which my equilibrium was off kilter. By the time we had stacked the plates in the sink and it looked like we might resume playing I was already like a cat on hot bricks.

The analogy was actually rather apt. Josh had two very cute Siamese kittens who padded around his flat like feline ninjas. Initially dubious of me, by the time I'd been sitting still for a while the braver of the two came up to sit on my lap. Being a sucker for pets generally, this made me smile, and before I knew it I'd been fussing him for a long while, chuckling at him cleaning my fingers with his sandpapery tongue. In what was, probably, slightly bad form, I wasn't hugely aware of where Josh was, until suddenly he was stroking the back of my neck, echoing the way I was fussing his cat. I shivered slightly underneath him, enjoying it, my body responding to – *finally!* – his touch. But then his fingers moved away and instead, he was running something up and down my spine. The drumstick. I froze.

The idea of a drumstick as a punishment implement came about because of a discussion about the plethora of computer games where you can now pretend to be a guitarist, vocalist or drummer in your own band. I made the mistake of arguing with him about them and turned out to be wrong, which in hindsight is entirely likely since I'd never played them while it turned out he was an expert. He decided that my punishment should be using a drumstick from the game. I had, through various other slips of the tongue, mainly brought about by being incapable of restraining my sarcastic streak, accrued 100 strikes with the drumstick, although I wasn't overly concerned – it was small, not especially bendy and I wasn't convinced he'd be able to get any kind of angle with which to cause me particular pain. That said, feeling him running it up and down my back made me fight to hide a shiver.

I sat stroking the cat, staring intently at his fur, listening to him purr as Josh stood behind me, stroking me. As the silence lengthened finally he moved in front of me, and plucked the cat from my lap, stroking him tenderly and rubbing his cheek against his face before putting him on the floor and taking my hand.

'I think it's time for us to leave the cats to it for the night.'

My throat was suddenly dry and the butterflies that had been in my stomach for the last two days started fluttering harder than ever. Never before had I felt such relief and such nerves at the same time. Finally this was going to happen. He led me to his bedroom.

The cats, it seemed, wanted to play too. As they followed us inside he picked them up one at a time and indulgently fussed them before gently, but firmly, leading them to the bedroom door, whispering to them and stroking behind their ears as he put them down in the hallway. It was so sweet to watch, and made the change in tone when he closed the door, turned to me and told me to strip feel even more incongruous. He sat down to watch as I began to take my clothes off.

Every woman, no matter how perfect, has parts of her body she's unhappy with, and trust me when I say I have a fair few imperfections. Generally, however, I try not to worry. I eat healthily, go to the gym at least three times a week, and am fairly optimistic that in the throes of passion most blokes are concerned about many many things that aren't whether your stomach's looking a bit flabby.

That said, being told to strip naked in front of someone you fancy who is (a) staying resolutely clothed and (b) thus not doing anything other than watching you intently as your remove your clothes is a very disconcerting thing. With an economy of movements and very little grace, I took my top off, pulled my trousers down – pulling my socks off at the same time, since they really are inherently unsexy – and then stayed still for a moment, screwing up my courage for the next step.

I looked at him looking at me, saw the smile playing at the corner of his mouth and decided it was time to play him at his own game. I could do this. I could fake a confidence I didn't feel. Hell, I had to do it for work sometimes, admittedly for non-naked reasons, and no one ever cottoned on. So smiling slightly, and hoping that I wasn't blushing as red as the heat from my face made me fear I was, I pulled my hands behind my back and undid my bra, pulling it forward and off. Not stopping I then went straight for my knickers, stacking both items on top of everything else on his bed. Then I turned back to him, resisting the urge to cross my arms across my chest with every fibre of my being.

We stayed that like for a few minutes. Me, with the breeze of the open window playing across my naked body, Josh sitting watching me. The early evening sunshine lit up the room and the sounds of car doors opening and closing and some kids playing football outside made it feel surreal. But still I stood there.

Finally he moved.

As he walked across the room and put his arm around me to cup my arse I curled into him, needing this, needing him. He leant down to kiss me and everything else melted away except feeling his hands on my body and his lips on mine. Then he pulled back, brushing a strand of my hair over my shoulder and smiled at me.

'Mmmmm. Before we do anything else you need to take your punishment. Do you remember what it was for?'

Apart from a couple of specific instances I couldn't remember the misdemeanours for my accrued punishments, however, I am not a complete idiot so I nodded yes. Thankfully this was enough.

'Good.' He led me across the room to a rug in front his fireplace. 'I'd like you to bend over, you can put your hands on your ankles or your knees, whichever is more comfortable. But once you're in position you stay there. You're going to count them for me and thank me for every strike. Is that clear?'

My voice was muffled by my long hair falling into my face as I assumed the position. 'Yes.'

He tapped me once on the arse in warning. 'Yes, sir.'

Then he began.

The first ten didn't hurt at all. I counted them off, thanking him for each one, calling him sir, generally not really bothered about the taps on my arse, thinking instead with anticipation about what would happen once we'd got this daft punishment out of the way.

Then suddenly something clicked – the angle he was using changed imperceptibly, or he found his rhythm, or something, and suddenly it hurt so much it took my breath away. I kept counting, stayed upright – just – although at one point he caught me with such force where my arse met my thigh that I stumbled slightly and had to use my hands to right myself. I did so quickly, apologising desperately lest he decide to add more for me moving from position. Fortunately he didn't.

With every stroke I thanked him, although by the time we reached fifty my teeth were gritted and my voice didn't sound very thankful at all. It hurt so much more than I had expected it to, and sheer bloody-mindedness was the only thing keeping me upright and counting. His rhythm was relentless, focusing purely on my left arse cheek, and as he kept hitting the same spot the pain began to build until I was finding it harder and harder to force any thanks from my dry throat.

At sixty he stopped for a moment. He grabbed a handful of hair and pulled my face up so he could look into my eyes.

'Are you crying? You sound like you're crying.'

The part of me that is all stubborn pride and no self-preservation answered before the rest of me could even think. 'I'm not.'

He looked closely, his eyes searching mine to assess how close he was to breaking me – something which actually made me feel safer and more calm, despite the pain I was processing. He nodded slightly at what he saw in my face. 'Do you need to stop?'

My chin raised and I heard my voice from far away sounding more assured than I felt. 'No. I'm fine.' What an idiot.

As he let go of my hair and moved behind me all I could think of was my mum's continual warning that stubbornness would one day be my downfall – although frankly I don't think this was exactly what she had in mind. He started on my arse again and – thankfully – thoughts of Mum disappeared as I began desperately trying to process the pain once more.

By the time we got to eighty it was all I could do to stand. I remained in position – a victory for pigheadedness – but with every stroke my inner monologue was screaming 'Twenty to go, nineteen to go, eighteen to go.' My legs were wobbling and I was in agony. When we got to a hundred the relief rushed through me. So much for the sodding drumstick not hurting that much.

Josh allowed me to stand upright and moved in front of me, kissing my forehead gently as I trembled in front of him, the pain and adrenaline thrumming through me.

'Good girl. Well done. You were very brave.'

I bit back a grimace at the hated endearment and he ran a finger along my cunt, the first time he ever had, and I moaned in pleasure, leaning into him and enjoying him exploring me with his fingers. He chuckled at how wet I was, how my legs started to shake as he pushed me – ridiculously easily – to the brink of orgasm. Then he pulled away. I managed to bite back a whimper – I had no intention of doing anything that would see him picking up the drumstick again – but I'm sure my eyes betrayed my frustration as he sat down on the edge of the bed, undoing his trousers and freeing his cock.

'Suck me.'

Oh. OK then. Definitely not a hardship.

I knelt down happily and opened my mouth to take him. I licked him greedily, loving the feeling of his hands in my hair, feeling him clench and unclench his fingers as I began to worship him with my mouth. I lost myself completely in the task, even the pain of my left arse cheek receding as I sucked him as deeply as I could into my mouth.

But then he pulled me away by my hair and took my arms to lift me up from my knees and back towards the rug. My brain actually short-circuited for a minute. I could see the direction he was trying to manoeuvre me in, and all I could think of was the drumstick and the pain. But I couldn't form words, much less sentences, and instead I heard myself making a desperate mewing noise from the back of my throat that was both a plea and a refusal. For a few seconds as he spoke to me I couldn't understand what he was saying such was the depth of my panic at being made to return to the punishment, but then as he kissed my forehead again and stroked me – with the same tenderness he'd shown his cats earlier – somehow I knew he was trying to alleviate my fears even through the rushing noise in my head. Finally I understood him.

'I'm not going to punish you again. I want you to stand over there so I can fuck you.'

Oh.

I let him help me to my feet and returned to the position I had been in a few minutes before. He rolled on a condom and began to fuck me, grabbing my hips to ensure he could fuck me as hard as possible, hitting my stinging arse with every thrust. It felt amazing. I was still on an adrenaline high from the punishment, I wasn't thinking about anything, I was just responding to him, reacting as he mastered me. As he reached round and began frigging my clit I came around him, my cries ringing loud in my ears although I was incapable of doing a bloody thing about it. After months of talking, weeks of anticipation, an evening of butterflies and the hardest and most unexpected punishment I'd received to date the intensity was just too much.

By the time I came back down to earth he had moved us both to the bed and I was lying (on my side, as putting any pressure on my arse was uncomfortable for at least the next week) alongside him. I looked up, suddenly a bit embarrassed at exactly how out of the moment I had gone, to see him smiling down at me. He stroked my hair and pressed another kiss to my forehead.

'You pleased me very well this evening. Good girl.'

I smiled, closing my eyes for a second to savour the gentleness of his lips. I can honestly say I wasn't bothered about the patronising tone now, instead all I felt was achievement, a kind of pride at having pleased him, the thought of a job well done.

Little did I realise this was just the beginning.

Chapter Nine

I PRIDE MYSELF ON not getting caught up in the clichéd etiquette of dating. Generally most of my friends are the same. There's none of this "these are the rules on when to call or not call" bollocks, we're all straightforward, sensible people. If you like someone what's the point in bullshitting?

So you'll never see me worrying about when I'm going to see someone again. If I want to see someone I'll ask. If they want to see me too then ace. If not, well, that's crap and my confidence'll take a knock, but I'll get over it.

Except it wasn't that way with Josh.

I'm honestly not hung up on gender stereotypes and try not to turn into that blithering cliché – *should I text, or is that too keen? If I text how many kisses should I put on the end? Hold on, he hasn't put a kiss on the end, but he did before, what does that mean?* But if I thought the etiquette of dating was bad, that's nothing to when you throw in a D/s power element to it. Is suggesting we meet again pushy? Unsubmissive? Should I be waiting for him to sort something? If he doesn't, do I just keep waiting? At what point should I give up and assume that actually he's not interested? Is the fact I'm the most impatient person I know likely to cause me a problem?

Meeting Josh coincided with the kind of time at work that made for a Kate of all work and no play. Various people were on holiday, a big launch of a new publication was in the works translating into the kind of hours that made sleeping under my desk seem like a tempting prospect as it meant I'd be getting more than six hours a night. All of which translated into me being a bit, well, disengaged. I talked to Josh by email pretty much every day, and found him as interesting as ever but over a period of a week or two things went from being steamy to, well, a bit tepid. I'd be bouncing work moans back and forth or linking him to stuff coming in on our newswire, but the smutty stuff? Somewhere along the way it dissipated in a way that left me thinking, *damn, obviously he's not as interested in me that way as I am in him*. So in characteristic fashion I decided the thing to do was to not address it, pretend everything was fine and leave it be. Until, erm, I couldn't any more and it burst forth like a slightly frightening torrent. Great.

It was a Thursday afternoon. The Thursday afternoon before The Big Project (TM) launched and the point in the process where everything seems insurmountable, except you know it'll be done because it has to be done and you'll just keep going until your eyes fall out of the back of your head and you can't think of another decent headline pun.

I was on Instant Messenger in part because I was discussing final colour choices for headers for the different sections of the magazine with our chief designer. But I'd been chatting to Josh in another window as he sat wrestling with some dry financial gubbins he had to turn into something readable.

The conversation had started incongruously enough but a passing comment that normally I'd have been sensible enough to leave alone started me off.

Josh says: We'll have to see what happens when we

next meet.

Kate says: Indeed. Although when will that be? Because we've yet to set anything up… :P

Ah, yes, a little jaunty tongue hides the neediness oozing from every syllable of that sentence. Oh dear. Must make it better.

Kate says: Not that I'm moaning.

Kate says: Just saying.

Kate says: And if you don't want to meet again – cause it has been a while now – then that's fine too. Really.

Shit, do I now sound like I'm not interested in him?

Kate says: I mean obviously I'd *like* to meet again.

Why is Vera Lynn running through my head now? How have I dug myself such a big bloody hole? How do I get out of it?

Kate says: But if you don't then that's fine, I'd just rather know.

Wow. You'd think it was difficult to sound both standoffish and needy at the same time, but I appeared to have managed it. Brilliant.

As I pondered whether disconnecting and blaming technical difficulties (and possibly partial lobotomy) was the best way of stopping this conversation without making it worse, I heard the ping of a response. I was fairly convinced it wouldn't be about whether green or purple best portrayed 'lifestyle' but could hardly bring myself to look at the screen to see.

Josh says: Of course I'd like to meet. What made you think I wouldn't?

Josh says: I just figured bearing in mind how stressed you sound every time I speak to you lately that looming over you like some überdom was perhaps not the most supportive course of action.

Josh says: I take it this is a subtle hint that you might

134

be free and inclined to play some time soon then?

Oh. Suddenly even the shittiest day at work wasn't bothering me at all and I caught myself grinning at the screen in a way which quite probably was terrifying my co-workers since it's the first time I'd cracked a smile in working hours for about a fortnight.

All of which is how I ended up spending a full 24 hours under Josh's control. At his suggestion I booked a day off work for the day after the big big project went to press – on time and with most of us still with our sanity intact. It was a great idea, as the morning after something comes out all you do is sit at your desk drinking coffee and praying the phone won't ring as, if it does, it's someone telling you something's gone wrong which you now can do nothing about anyway. So spending a day alone with him, not knowing exactly what would happen, and burning off some excess energy was an idea that sounded relaxing and brilliant. At least it did until I realised exactly what I'd let myself in for, and that "relaxing" was never in a million years going to be an adjective to describe it.

I arrived at 7.30pm after a schlep through the rush-hour traffic, and any curiosity about how this would all start was ended rather abruptly. I followed him into his flat, bending down to pet the cats hello. As I stood up, I swapped my overnight bag to my other hand. As his eyes took it in, he moved towards me, plucking it from my grasp.

'You won't be needing that,' he told me as he led me into the living room, chucking it on the floor. He plonked himself down on the sofa and I stood in front of him, awkward, not entirely sure what to do as he was sprawled across it in a way so there was no space for me. At least I was unsure until he spoke, and then it all made sense.

'Strip for me. Now.'

I looked at him, relaxed and smiling like someone in a sofa commercial, secure in the knowledge that I was going to do what he asked. As ever, the beginning of a scene remained the most difficult part for me and the picture of arrogance he made lying there waiting for me to move, knowing that it was inevitable I would, made me grit my teeth as I slipped out of my shoes and began undoing my shirt.

'Hold on a second, stop.'

My hands stopped on my third button at his order. I looked over at him, wishing he'd make up his mind – did he want me to undress or not?

'Yes?' My voice sounded a bit shrill to my own ears, I knew it was from embarrassment, but worrying that he might interpret it as attitude I lowered my tone. 'Sir?'

His eyes sparkled as he spoke to me, inspiring a surge of affection even while it caused butterflies in the pit of my stomach. Butterflies which started going mad at what he said next.

'For the next 24 hours you are mine. Mine only. Everything you do is for me. Your wishes, your needs, even your dignity, count for nothing. You will do everything I ask you to do, to the best of your ability, in the way which you know will bring me the most pleasure. Is that clear?'

I had to swallow hard before I could speak. The immediate ramifications of this had already started running through my mind, and a blush was beginning to stain my cheeks. 'Yes, sir.'

'Well then, don't you think you should slow down and take your clothes off in a way that you know will please me?'

I didn't trust myself to speak, so nodded.

'Good girl. Well then, strip for me. Not functionally, sensually. Show me your body. Show me my property.'

While intellectually I knew he was pushing me to see a reaction, it took a lot of effort not to push back, particularly at the idea of being his "property", even though I knew that was effectively the deal we had done, and that – actually – there was a great part of me keen to surrender to him in that way for a little while to see where he took us.

My teeth were gritted and my fingers clumsy as I began playing with my partially open top, flashing a glimpse of my bra as I ran my hands down my body, over my hips and skirt before slowly beginning to undress once more.

The five minutes that followed felt like an eternity. If it wasn't for the fact that I spent a great part of the time too embarrassed to look at Josh and instead staring over his shoulder, looking at the wall behind him which happened to have a clock on it, I'd have sworn it went on for nearer an hour.

I'm comfortable in my own skin, but I'm both aware my body is far from perfect and not the kind of person who likes being the centre of attention at the best of times. Being made to strip in that way made me feel ridiculous, embarrassed, objectified. Every instinct was telling me to get it over with quickly, even while I knew I had to take my time, tease and tantalise as well as I could.

By the time I was down to my knickers an embarrassed flush had bloomed across my chest as well as my face, and I was hiding behind my hair as much as possible. I don't think I had ever felt as vulnerable and the feeling was prickly, unpleasant. My throat felt clogged and I was inexplicably close to tears.

I finally pulled down my knickers and stood in front of him, naked, physically and emotionally. After long seconds he moved towards me.

'Your posture really is atrocious you know.'

His face was unreadable as he leant around me, his hands reaching around my back to push my shoulder blades, making my breasts stand out, the nipples rubbing against the rough wool of his jumper.

'I know it's because you feel embarrassed about the size of your tits,' – at that he ran a finger along the line of fire across my chest – 'but there really is no excuse for it and hunching over doesn't make them look smaller. You shouldn't be hiding them anyway.'

I felt shy, which was ridiculous. My voice sounded unlike me to my ears. 'Sorry.'

He tutted, tweaking a nipple in rebuke.

'I see we're also going to have to work on ensuring you use the correct modes of address as well.' Shit.

'Sorry. Sir.'

He smiled and the queasy feeling in my stomach disappeared, replaced with a pride that was as shocking as it was warming. Knowing I'd pleased him made the awkwardness seem somehow worthwhile. Although the sooner he ended up naked too, the happier I knew I'd be.

He smoothed my hair away from my face as I stood still, waiting for what came next. But he kissed my shoulder and then moved behind me.

I could hear sounds of rummaging, a cupboard door opening, and then a jangling sound that made me want to turn around even though I knew I shouldn't. I stood, shoulders back, waiting nervously for whatever was to happen next.

He was back in front of me, not carrying anything to have me running for the hills. In fact, not actually carrying anything at all that I could see.

'Do you trust me?'

'Yes.' My answer was quick, firm and sure. I honestly did.

The last thing I saw was his smile as he pulled a blindfold he'd had scrunched in one of his hands over my eyes.

'Good.'

Never having been blindfolded during sex before, or, come to think of it, for anything other than a few games of blind man's buff at birthday parties as a child, I was surprised at how vulnerable I felt.

Having deliberately avoided his gaze during my strip tease just minutes earlier, being in a position where I couldn't see anything didn't make me feel less embarrassed or shy, it just made me feel more exposed. And of course meant I had even less idea about what would happen next.

I waited.

The jangling was back and he was behind me, grabbing my wrists, cuffing them in something that felt cold and unyielding. Then my ankles were tied together with something tighter, something fabric, that gave me a tiny bit of shuffle room but not much else.

I felt him straighten up behind me, although his voice whispering directly into my ear made me jump.

'I think we're going to work on your posture now, sweet. I know you feel embarrassed showing yourself to me, but right now that's all I want from you. I'm going to get a glass of wine and sit down and just admire you for a little bit, while I decide what I'm going to do to you next.'

His teeth nipped my ear and he chuckled as I shivered. 'So many possibilities. So many ideas. I just don't know where to start. Get down on your knees.'

Dropping to your knees when your ankles are tied together and your hands are behind you makes you more off balance, so getting down to the floor took a little while and left me feeling rather ungainly.

I'd lost track of where he was in the room, couldn't even be sure he hadn't popped to the kitchen for his wine, and yet still felt like his eyes were on me. Finally I got to my knees, pulled my shoulders back to push my breasts out and sat and waited.

And waited.

Every movement and change of air in the room made me start. Was that him? Was that one of the cats? And if so how the hell was I going to shoo them away?

Suddenly his hand was in my hair and his voice back in my ear, making me jump.

'Spread your legs for me. I want to see you.'

I shuffled on the carpet, opening my knees a little.

His tut – now in front of me – made me start, and I felt his foot push at my knee, making me spread myself wider in wanton fashion.

'That's better. I want to see how wet treating you like this makes you, even in spite of yourself. You are looking quite aroused already and I've not even touched you yet. You're flushed – but I'm not sure it's embarrassment anymore, although God knows it should be, you filthy slut. Instead I think you're turned on. Your nipples look like they're aching for my touch, or my teeth. And as for your cunt. You're glistening.'

Suddenly I was very glad for the blindfold as I knew, despite – or perhaps because of – my uncomfortableness, he was right. I could feel the heavy wetness between my legs.

He pushed me yet wider with his foot and I wondered

140

fleetingly why I didn't feel the fury I would normally. The bonds, the blindfold, something has changed the dynamic and it felt unreal. Hyperreal. Something.

'Your juice is on my shoe. Dirty girl. I should make you lick it off. If you make a mess you should clean it up. It's only fair, right?'

OK, the fury was back. I didn't argue, but my tone was more mutinous than I'd have liked as I replied. 'Whatever you wish, sir.'

He laughed. 'Good answer. And I do like the idea of your tongue on my shoes, licking off the evidence of your arousal. But right now I'm liking looking up between your legs best of all.'

Even behind the blindfold I closed my eyes. I heard him take a drink – of his wine, I assumed.

He told me how he'd been pondering for months what it would be like to push me. How all the messages back and forth, the relatively sedate dinner, the initial play date had all been leading to this. How I didn't know what was going to hit me, had no idea what I'd let myself in for, that I was his now. And while I knew he was in the moment, and that I could trust him, fear cramped my stomach just a little as I couldn't move, I couldn't see. Suddenly I wished the blindfold was off, that I could look into his eyes for a moment and see the reassurance there. As it was, I just felt myself get a little panicky, and yet more aroused at the feeling of powerlessness.

I knelt in silence, my lips pressed together to stop them trembling, waiting to see what would happen next. I felt his eyes on me – I think – and every movement in the room made me shrink slightly, waiting for a touch, something.

I heard him take another drink and my throat felt suddenly dry. I swallowed.

'Are you thirsty?' he asked, from the direction of the sofa. 'Would you like something to drink?'

I nodded and then thought better of it. 'Yes, please.' He didn't respond, and after a few seconds I realised why. Dammit. 'Sir.'

I felt him leaning towards me. 'Good girl. I'm tempted to fill a bowl with some water and see if I can tempt you to drink from it like an animal–' suddenly I thought I could manage without a drink for now and something in my demeanour must have betrayed how unhappy I was with this suggestion as he laughed at my reaction '–but I'll be kind this time.'

He pushed a glass to my lips. I put my mouth round it tentatively, wondering suspiciously for a moment what it was, before he tilted it and I had to swallow or have it pour down my front.

It was soda water with ice and some lemon, and it tasted amazing, although as he tilted the glass further and I had to drink faster to avoid wearing it, I felt a surge of anger at the fact he was demonstrating his power over me with even the simplest of things.

He moved back to the sofa, and I heard the crunch of him eating something. My position, the fact that seemingly I was some kind of blind floorshow while he had a snack made me furious. Thank goodness I had the blindfold on to hide it.

'Are you all right there, sweet? Is there something you want to say?'

I wasn't hiding it well then. I knew he was trying to get a rise out of me, and you'd think that knowing that would have made it easier to keep a feeling of zen-like calm. It's wasn't.

'No, thank you. I'm fine.'

He stroked my hair.

'If you're sure. I'd hate for you to feel you couldn't speak freely.'

I knew that speaking freely would get me into lots of trouble so I shook my head and pressed my lips together to avoid the urge.

'Are you hungry? Is that the problem? Would you like me to feed you?'

Mindful of his threat to have me drinking from a bowl, I had no intention of eating food in a similar way, definitely a debasement too far. I opened my mouth to say no, and his fingers were at my lips, pushing something in. A cube of some kind of cheese. I chewed it slowly, enjoying it. As I swallowed his fingers were back, this time with an olive. Oily, sweet. As I swallowed, his fingers were back at my mouth, empty this time. Without thinking I sucked them into my mouth and licked them clean. So much for not being demeaned or treated like some kind of animal. Suddenly I felt like one of his cats.

He pulled his fingers away and he was pushing at my mouth again, although this time it was his cock he was pressing to my lips. I opened my mouth to welcome him, eager, enjoying sucking him, until he grabbed me by the hair, holding me in place as he began fucking my mouth. I wriggled my arms for a second, the panic of beginning to feel choked making me forget that I couldn't move my hands round to do anything. I was snuffling round his cock, desperately trying to breathe, twisting my head to try and pull back, just a little. I felt him thicken in my mouth at my struggles, making it worse, and I tried to signal somehow that this was too much, that he needed to give me a second. Except I couldn't gesture, couldn't speak and while the blindfold was wet with my tears I wasn't entirely sure he was aware of that. Or actually that he cared.

When he came in my mouth I swallowed him as well as I could, although as he pulled out I gasped to catch my breath and I felt something – either his spunk or my drool – dripping down my chin. Classy.

He tugged on my hair, and I half crawled, half shuffled across the floor as best I could in my bonds, moving closer to the sofa, so he could stroke my hair as he sat down. I calmed a little, my heartbeat slowing, although I still felt well and truly on the back foot.

I don't know how long we sat there, but it was long enough for our breathing to slow. His hand on my hair was almost hypnotic and I was soothed as we sat quietly. Until he spoke again.

'We still have to work on your posture. And your modes of address. Don't we?'

Bugger. Where's this coming from? How many times had I not called him sir in the last hour? And how bad had the slouching been? I pushed my shoulders back, closing the stable door after the horse has bolted? Possibly. But it couldn't hurt could it?

He tweaked my nipple, bringing me out of my panic. 'Don't we?'

'Yes.'

'Yes?'

Gah.

'Yes, sir.'

He pulled me to my feet and freed my arms. I stretched a little, feeling happier and slightly more in control – for half a second, until he refastened them in front of me.

'Bend over.'

My heart was pounding already as this posture was Josh's preferred punishment stance.

Shit.

His voice was in my ear. Harsh in a way that probably

would have been less intimidating if I could see him, but made me feel a jolt of genuine fear.

'I won't tell you again. Bend over.'

I trembled as I moved into position, but I didn't think of disobeying. Was this progress or stupidity? I wasn't entirely sure. He started hitting me, not with the drumstick but with something else. Something longer, with more give and which hurt so much that the air rushed out of my lungs with every strike in time with the swooshing noise of it cutting the air and connecting with my arse.

He hit one cheek, and then the other. There was no rhythm to it, nothing to count, no indication of how long it would last. I have no idea how many times he hit me, just that it hurt, it hurt so damn much. I'd never felt pain like it. Each strike hurt, and the feeling of the residual strikes was like a burning agony, layer upon layer of pain as he kept going. It made Sarah's punishment seem feather-light in comparison, and not knowing how long this would last made it feel impossible to bear.

Finally he stopped. His hand squeezing my arse made me suck air in through my teeth.

'Do you think you'll remember now?'

My reply was garbled, desperate, quick. 'Yes. Yes. Definitely.'

Quick and stupid. I realised the error as he moved away again.

'Sorry. Sir. Yes, sir.'

He began again. The strikes were faster than I could process. Faster than I could endure. Each one cut across my arse leaving a line of agony. I was sure I was bleeding, I couldn't imagine withstanding this amount of pain without it drawing blood.

I wanted to stop. But I didn't want to disappoint him. I

didn't want to use a safe word. I could withstand it. Not just out of stubborn bloody-minded pride, but because this was the most challenging thing we had ever done and I didn't intend to fail it. But it hurt so much and I had no idea how long it would last and I just couldn't cope. After the stresses and strains of the last few weeks at work, the humiliation and embarrassment of stripping earlier, the sensory deprivation that meant I couldn't even look to him for reassurance, it was all too much.

I started to cry, snotty, guttural sobbing. I couldn't stop myself. The noise sounded alien, shocking, even to my own ears. I sounded broken, desperate, wounded. He hit me a couple more times, and then I heard the clatter of whatever it was he was hitting me with landing on the floor. It had stopped. But I couldn't. I cried as he undid my wrists and ankles, pulled the blindfold from my eyes, grabbed a blanket from somewhere I didn't see. I cried as he led me to the sofa where he sat, patting his lap and encouraging me to curl up next to him putting my head on his thigh. I cried as he gently draped the blanket over my nakedness, making sure not to touch my arse as he did so. I cried until my throat was raw, until my sobs dissipated into snuffles and an occasional hiccup. I cried until I felt like I couldn't cry any more. They were tears of catharsis, release of a tension that I didn't even know I was carrying. I felt broken down and rebuilt. They weren't tears of upset, but I couldn't stop them. So I cried, and through it all he just stroked my hair and waited.

And then I fell asleep.

I woke up in a puddle of my own drool. On his thigh. Classy. He must have thought I was a complete nutjob all things considered. In a split second everything that had come before flashed through my mind and I was horrified.

I couldn't remember the last time I had made such a complete twat of myself and I felt stupid, and embarrassed and tearful and sick. I wanted to fling on my clothes and run away and not ever look at him again, but doing that would have involved moving and that would have involved speaking and having him look at me. So I lay very still in the flickering light of the TV that appeared to have been switched on at some point while I slept, trying to figure out what time it was and what on earth to do next.

'Are you awake?'

His voice was solicitous, neither laughing nor seemingly concerned about the fact he'd invited a nutter into his home who has jiggled about in unalluring fashion and nearly choked to death on his cock, before having a kind of panic attack and then passing out on his leg in a tidal wave of dribble.

The urge to feign sleep was strong but I figured he must have had his suspicions since he'd asked about ten seconds after I woke up. This probably meant I had been snoring on top of everything else. God, I could never see this man again.

My voice was quiet. 'No.'

He laughed and the vibrations of it make me jiggle slightly on his leg.

He stroked my hair and I felt warmed by the connection.

''No, sir'. Surely?'

Fuck. I went to sit up, desperate to set things straight before he started up again with whatever the hell that was. In my haste I managed to bash my arse with my foot and it hurt so much I whimpered. I was apologising, saying 'sir' every other word, desperate, giddy, horrified, looking into his face with pleading eyes for reassurance.

He stopped me with a single finger to my mouth. He was smiling, kind.

'Sssssssh. It's OK. It's OK. Your training is a work in progress. And you did very well. For now.'

He kissed me and adjusted the blanket so it covered us both better.

I think that was the moment when I started to fall in love with him.

Chapter Ten

AFTER THAT NIGHT JOSH and I settled into the typical first flushes of an almost relationship. By unspoken agreement we didn't define it, perhaps because subconsciously we felt that actually to do so might make the magic dissipate like early morning mist, but we had a lot of fun. We spoke every day, either by phone or email, texting at odd little moments when that didn't feel enough. We saw lots of films, walked by the river, spent hours talking over wine and cheese in a subterranean wine bar that felt like a different world from the hustle and bustle of London and generally did the sort of things that would be at home in the depiction of a burgeoning relationship in a chick flick. Except for the bit at the end where we'd go back to one or other of our homes and fuck and suck and bite and play until we were both exhausted and I was bruised and whimpering. Don't get me wrong, we weren't joined at the hip. I still saw Russell, both for smutty and unsmutty fun, although I found myself questioning whether this would continue. I'd even had the beginnings of a couple of conversations with him about potentially friends-zoning each other although, obviously, this didn't count as a new relationship. Yet. Well that's what I kept telling myself, despite thinking of Josh throughout the day like a lovestruck teenager and getting to the point where my first instinct when it came to talking about my day or sharing something great that had happened was to ring or text him. For six weeks we were almost permanently connected, constantly always just a few moments from speaking. And then I had to go away for work.

Hot on the heels of The-Big-Project-that-by-some-miracle-had-not-turned-into-a-catastrophe, I was asked to go and spend a week visiting another part of the company I work for, based in a different part of the country, to help them launch something similar. In typical journalistic fashion it meant long days and late nights, all of which meant I didn't hear from Josh anywhere near as much as I had been. I missed him – not just for the smut, actually – although my days were so packed that I found his absence made me especially wistful lying in bed at night when my mind finally had time to wander. But life was so busy that I didn't get to speak to him much, and I certainly didn't get a chance to write him the explicit fantasy of what we'd be doing the first night we were reunited that I'd promised to email while I was away. Frankly, hunched over my laptop for work for ten hours a day meant by the time I got back to the hotel room – invariably after a few glasses of red and some war stories and gossip with colleagues about friends of friends from the incestuous world of journalism – I just wasn't in the mindset to write anything sexy. And by the final night of my stay I'd figured it'd be enough I'd be seeing him shortly for us to be reacquainted in person, particularly since having asked about it a couple of times on the phone and by text he hadn't mentioned it since.

He rang not long after I'd got in from the pub. Freshly showered, I was curled up in bed with *Newsnight* on low when his name flashed up on my phone. I answered with a smile in my voice, which dimmed slightly when I heard his tone. While he answered my questions about how his day had gone, told me his cats' latest escapades, and asked politely about my launch, he was brusque in a way that left me feeling vaguely uneasy.

I soon found out why.

Normally our silences were easy but as the static on the line echoed in my ear and I waited for him to say something I couldn't think of anything to fill the void. It was obvious from the fact he'd rung that he wanted to talk about something specific, but waiting for him to do so was excruciating. In the long seconds I waited I had a sick feeling in the pit of my stomach, knowing how important a part of my life he had become in such a short period of time, and wondering how I would cope with the grief at the loss of this undefined relationship, if that was what he was gearing up to. Although how could he end it? We hadn't even defined it yet, damn it.

Finally he spoke. 'Do you have anything you want to tell me?'

My mind froze up for a second and suddenly I felt guilt-ridden. I know, it's ridiculous, I'd done nothing wrong that I could think of, but I still felt worried. What did he think I had to tell him? What had I done? Was this about my continuing to play with Russell? But we hadn't even discussed being exclusive and he knew all about it, had in fact been playing an impromptu game with Russell based on leaving exotic and impressive-looking marks on my body for the other to find in a way which amused both of them immensely even while I mocked them both for their competitiveness. It couldn't be that. What else could it be? I was one of the most boring people I knew – the closest thing to a secret I had was the D/s aspect of my life, and he knew all about that. My heart was racing but I had no idea what I was supposed to say and the knowledge of my ignorance made me feel completely powerless – and not in the kind of way that would normally make me wet.

'Well?' I didn't think his voice in my ear could get even more irritable, but it most definitely did.

I took a deep breath and went to speak but, honestly, I had nothing. I let the breath out and tried to at least sound calm. 'Like what? Is everything OK?'

Seconds ticked by. 'Do you think everything's OK, Kate?'

Shit. What did he mean by everything? Everything in the world? Everything in our non-relationshippy relationship? Everything we'd talked about today? I needed clues, something so I didn't feel this bloody tentative. 'I think so. Why? Do you not? Has something happened?'

His response was quick. 'No, Kate, nothing's happened, which is rather my point.'

I like to think on a normal day when my head wasn't fuzzy with a couple of glasses of wine, and the rising concern of him using my name twice in quick succession – one thing I'd learned with Josh was that this was a sign of impending trouble – I'd have got it then. Of course on this occasion I didn't, which was my eventual downfall.

'What do you mean?'

'What do you think I mean, Kate?' Three Kates. This was bad. And I still had no clue.

I tried to tamp down the sound of my frustration as I knew that would just makes things worse, but it was touch and go. I bit the words out – this kind of powerlessness makes me want to kick things. 'I don't know, that's why I'm asking.'

He sighed, and I felt a pang at annoying him, in spite of the fact he was fast annoying me to the point I wished I'd just not picked up the phone when he rang and told him later I was asleep. 'What was the one thing you were supposed to do this week, Kate?'

Oh. Bugger. He hadn't forgotten. Of course not.

'The email, of course, the email. I'm sorry I haven't got round to it, it's just work's been so mad, the net connection at the hotel's rubbish, I've not been feeling especially sexy and, well, I'm just so tired every night –' I tailed off, my voice sounding whiny even to myself.

His voice was so quiet that I had to put a finger to my other ear to block out the world to hear it. 'I asked you to do one thing Kate. Have you done it?'

Suddenly I had a lump in my throat and an odd ache in my heart and I wished with every fibre of my being that I had a different answer for him. And this wasn't playing, wasn't fun, was about me feeling bad for having let him down, for – perhaps – having inadvertently hurt him by not doing something to prove I'd been thinking of him while I'd been away, and for not obeying him in the way I should have. My voice was quiet. 'No. I haven't. I'm sorry.'

There was no noise on the line but static, and as I listened to it the feeling of guilt at letting him down weighed on me.

'I put something into the side pocket of your overnight bag. Go and get it.'

I don't know what I was expecting when I opened the brown paper bag, but my trepidation dissipated when I pulled out four pairs of chopsticks not unlike those you'd get at your local Chinese takeaway.

'So what have you got?'

I couldn't hide the bemusement in my voice. 'Chopsticks. Enough for a bit of a feast actually.'

He chuckled and for a moment he was my Josh and

even though he was pissed off I felt a little less worried. And then he was back to business. 'You'll need three pairs, and the rubber bands.'

Rubber bands? I dug them out of the bottom of the bag. Hmmm.

'Wind a rubber band round each end of each of the three pairs. Tightly.' I began doing so, unsure exactly about where this was going to go, but trying to make amends by, admittedly, shutting the stable door after the horse of obedience had well and truly bolted. 'And when you've done that strip naked.'

Oh.

His voice in my ear was reasonable. There was no anger, not even his earlier pique. He sounded resolute yet calm. What was about to happen was inevitable. It might or might not give him pleasure, but that was academic, it had to be done, as a lesson. I knew this before he said it, as I heard him explain how, in a moment I was going to punish myself.

To be honest I wasn't entirely sure how that would work, bearing in mind I am such a wuss when it comes to inflicting pain on myself. I don't pluck my own eyebrows because it hurts too much. Still, on the plus side, how hard could it be? Anything that I did on myself was going to be significantly lighter-handed than Josh would be had he been here in person. Right? Of course, I underestimated him. As he explained to me how I was to trap each of my nipples between these impromptu chopstick clamps I realised that it wasn't simple as I thought. And then he told me to put the first one on.

For a split second before the bands holding the chopsticks together snapped back into place I thought it would be all right. More proof, if any were needed, that I am in fact an idiot. It hurt. A lot. I pushed air through my

154

nose, trying to process the pain by breathing deeply, riding it, waiting desperately for the change to a dull ache as my nipple became numb rather than the excruciating fire. By the time it did my breathing was ragged and I was trying not to cry.

Finally I trusted myself to speak. 'It's on.'

'Really? That's interesting. I didn't realise you were telepathic. Are you a fucking mind reader then, Kate?'

'What?' I actually couldn't focus on what he was saying, the pain in my nipple was so acute.

'Did you ask me which way round I wanted you to place the clamp?'

Bugger it. 'No, no I didn't.'

'Silly, silly girl. Which way round did you put it?'

I could see where this was going and I was filled with both trepidation and fury. I answered, my tone mutinous, made so by the knowledge that whichever way it was it wasn't going to be right. 'It's horizontal across my breast.'

He tutted loudly in a way that made me grateful we weren't in the same room as I knew I wouldn't be able to stop myself glaring at him, which would have just got me into more trouble. 'Oh dear. If only you'd asked me first. I want it running diagonally towards your shoulder. Twist it round. Now.'

The small voice in the back of my mind that does a running commentary throughout my submission was asking me why on earth I was acquiescing to this agony, so far away, when Josh couldn't even see me. But the larger part of me wanted to please him, to make amends, to be brave, to make him proud. And I was going to do exactly that, as soon as I stopped my hands shaking.

I had to pull the chopsticks apart for a second before I could twist the clamp around. Releasing my nipple caused a surge of agonising sensation. I couldn't stop my whimper even as it snapped back into place.

He murmured in approval. 'Good girl. Now put the second one on.'

'Which way round do you want it?' I couldn't stop myself from snapping.

Thankfully he laughed, ignoring my tone. 'Good question. Symmetrical to the first. Do it right and you won't have to move it.'

I picked up the second set of chopsticks and pulled them apart, steeling myself for the pain.

I had been lying on the bed, naked and unmoving, for about ten minutes when he spoke again. Having put the second pair of chopsticks on, and then the third, it was all I could do to lie quietly holding the phone listening to him breathing gently a few hundred miles away. My breathing was, in comparison, ragged. I hadn't cried out again, I was focused on dealing with the pain, watching distantly as the chopstick clamps rose and fell with each breath.

Putting the chopsticks on my other nipple caused more trepidation than the first one, because I knew how much it hurt. My nipples were taut, red, hurting with a pulsating pain which came in throbbing waves. As for my clit, the poor recipient of the third and final set of chopsticks, it was engorged, sore and aching, held tightly in place between my spread-out legs.

I lay there trying my hardest not to move, not to do anything that would exacerbate the pain thrumming through my body. Enduring it, knowing I owed Josh this, trying to withstand it, determined not to let him down again. And then I nearly dropped the phone when he said: 'Right. Now I think it's time for us to start your punishment Kate, don't you?'

Start? Oh hell.

His voice in my ear was charming, reasonable. He didn't sound angry, just matter of fact about the fact that he'd known I wouldn't get round to writing my assignment, that for someone whose professional life depended so much on deadlines I was a procrastinator, leaving things till the last minute or letting them slide completely. He told me how he'd slipped the chopsticks in the side pocket of my bag the last night we'd seen each other, hoping he wouldn't need to use them. How he'd asked me about how the writing was going in the hope I'd have done some, and become increasingly disappointed with me when it became apparent that not only was I not bothering but that I was flippantly dismissing his questions about when it would be done. How it showed a lack of respect he couldn't allow.

I lay there, my body aching, listening to him intently, filled with remorse at disappointing him, waiting for my chance to apologise. Except then he asked me how wet I was. I didn't know what to say. Even with the agony pinched around my clit – I was thankful the nipples had eased to a dull ache as the minutes lengthened – I knew I was wet. But this was punishment after all. Should I admit that to him? Or would that make it worse? While my pain-addled brain wrestled with the conundrum – was it worse to lie or worse to admit the truth? – he chuckled.

'Don't worry pet, I know you are. You can't help it, in spite of yourself, can you?'

I made a noise of disagreement in the back of my throat, and then, frankly, thought better of it.

'Slip a finger between your legs. Cover your clit with your juice. Can you do that?'

I moved tentatively, frightened of knocking one of the sets of chopsticks at my breasts. I pushed a finger inside my now slick folds and began rubbing my clit, moving it slightly within its chopstick prison in a way which hurt, but – in spite of myself – beginning to enjoy the delicious sensation merging with the pain. But as my breathing changed, betraying me, Josh firmly told me to stop. I restrained a whimper of frustration – I thought it was safest under the circumstances, and I was definitely right as it turned out.

'What am I punishing you for, girl?'

'For not sending you the email I promised. I'm so sorry.'

'You will be, I promise you that. But that's not all. What else?'

Shit. What else? What else had I done? I honestly couldn't think of anything more but if I said that and was wrong …

As I tried desperately to think of what he could be referring to he tutted in my ear. 'You don't even remember it, do you?' My heart started to pound. 'Not only did you not do what I asked – the one small thing in amongst everything else you've been doing this last week – but I asked you on three separate occasions whether you were doing it and three times you told me you were. On one notable occasion you sent me a text where you blew a raspberry –' his voice was incredulous at the idea I would dare do such a thing, '– at me for implying that you wouldn't do what I had asked you to.'

Oh God. I started to apologise again but he cut me off. 'I don't want you to speak until I tell you to. Frankly I don't trust any of the words that come tripping off your tongue. Which leads me to your punishment.'

Leads him to? If I had the breath I would probably have asked him what the fuck everything up to this point was. With hindsight it's better that I didn't.

'Take the clamp off your clit. Now.'

I was relieved at his order, thankful that whatever I was to endure at least wouldn't involve the throbbing agony of my clit too. My hands moved eagerly and although my gasp as I pulled the clamp clear was loud, I remained silent as the blood returned to my poor tortured clit, making me squirm on the bed at the increased pain.

The change in my breathing didn't go unnoticed. 'Good girl.' I felt warmed by his praise, even in the middle of his punishment, and it meant I was lulled into a false sense of security. 'Now take that clamp and put it around your tongue.'

The security vanished like mist and I couldn't stay silent. 'What?'

'You heard me. Your lying tongue has got you into this mess, and it's going to get its part of your punishment. Stick your tongue out and put the chopsticks around it. As far back as you can. Now. Clamp it for me.'

My hands were shaking. I was furious. Embarrassed. Guilty. Shy. Wondering why the fuck I was letting him do this, but knowing that I would, that this would be my penance. Not knowing how much it would hurt made me feel queasy with fear, but I knew I owed him it, just hoped I could do this. Yes, I'd look stupid, but no one would be able to see. And Josh wouldn't be able to hear me. It'd be fine. I could do this. I could.

I did it.

The first thing I was aware of as the impromptu clamp closed around my tongue was the taste of my juice. A split second later the sensation caught up and I felt a surge of pain. I whimpered, and I honestly wouldn't have been able to say which feeling was more upsetting – well actually I wouldn't have been able to say anything. I tried to roll the chopsticks along my tongue a little, so they would settle comfortably between my teeth, like a bit for a wayward horse.

'Is it on?'

Stupidly I nodded before murmuring my assent.

'I bet you can taste yourself can't you, you filthy slut?'

I know he expected an answer but my second murmur was quieter and – if it's possible to for a murmur to sound that way – filled with shame.

He laughed. 'Come on now, Kate. You know the rules. Answer me properly.'

I was furious. I clamped my lips round the chopsticks as well as I could when my tongue was sticking out into the night air.

'You can speak with a clamp like that on, Kate, and you will speak. I've got all night and all you're doing is causing more problems for yourself.'

I stayed silent.

'Right. Slap your cunt. Hard. Three times.'

I hated it when he has me do this, mainly because he was insistent it has to be loud enough to hear down the phone. My hand was clenching and unclenching above my head while I screwed up enough courage to inflict the first blow. I slapped myself, harder than I meant to, catching my clit. I accidentally bit my tongue trying to stifle a moan. The second blow was fine – if vicious self-torture can ever be described as fine – but the third was agony as I managed to knock the clamp around my left nipple as I moved my hand down. I couldn't stop myself crying out and I heard a tut in my ear for my trouble. The sound of his tuts were seriously beginning to piss me off even as I struggled to obey him.

'You're rude tonight, Kate, as well as disobedient. You know you should thank me for every blow I inflict on you.'

I couldn't speak. I wouldn't speak. And then he said something to fill me with a terror I couldn't quell.

'We can keep on at this all night. You're now going to slap your cunt six times. And if you don't count them off and thank me for each blow then I am going to double it, and double that, and we are going to keep going until you give me what I want. So it's entirely up to you. I'm happy to lie here all evening listening to your snuffling desperation, it's quite entertaining actually. But one way or another you are going to take your punishment. And you are going to speak to me.'

In that moment I hated him. This wasn't about submitting to feel challenged, or be aroused or even to arouse him. He wasn't pushing me out of my comfort zone or humiliating me for our mutual pleasure. But he was humiliating me, demeaning me, in a way he never had before. I properly hated him, but the loathing was tinged with prickly embarrassment and a genuine feeling of guilt. I opened my mouth to try and speak, tried to form words around my immobile tongue, tried to swallow back some of the drool pooling at the corners of my mouth. It was like standing on the edge of the precipice. I knew what he wanted. Knew the choice was mine. Knew actually that I didn't want to do it, that my every instinct was shouting for me not to, that I should hang up. But I wanted to make amends. I wanted to please him. I wanted to be able to reach the bar he had raised rather than failing him, failing myself. The choice was mine. In a way I hated that it was, as it made the submission, the humiliation more acute, more distressing. The choice was mine, and I was choosing to take this punishment, to be demeaned this way, and what's more he knew I was going to, even as he knew how much I was hating every second of it.

I slapped my cunt. Hard enough that I gasped at the impact. And then, stiltedly, my voice thick with tears, I managed to say: 'One. Thank you.'

Actually I didn't. I said something that sounded ridiculous. Lisping and unintelligible except for the fact it was the right number of syllables. Probably. I felt a surge of shame and humiliation, and, trying to ignore it, I slapped my cunt again. Hearing myself speak a second time was actually worse than the first, although I can't exactly explain why. I still sounded like an idiot and as I heard myself, how ridiculous and debased I sounded, I started to cry, becoming even less intelligible. I kept slapping and counting and thanking (although I'm not sure how thankful I actually came across) and by the time I got to six I was sobbing, hoping this unlikely indignity would soon be over.

Punishments are funny things. A lot of the D/s dynamic is about pain – inflicting it, withstanding it. But being spanked or caned for some spurious play reason is fun, makes me wet. This was different. I felt so sorry for having disappointed him, sad that he had seen it as inevitable to the extent he had pre-packed punishment implements, and suddenly, lying on a hotel bed far from home, with aching nipples and a sore tongue being made to do demeaning and horrifying things, I felt awful and alone. And yes, I appreciate that's what a punishment should do. I just wasn't expecting six chopsticks and a dozen rubber bands to do the job so well.

After a little while I was able to slow my tears, tentatively trying to brush them away without knocking any chopsticks. My sobs switched to the occasional snuffle and finally he spoke.

'Do you understand why I've punished you this way?'

I swallowed round the chopsticks the best I could

before lisping my 'yes', shutting my eyes at the ridiculous sound I made.

'I have punished you like this because you've been a silly little girl and this is how silly little girls get punished.' If I was being my normal smart-arsed self I'd have said something then, or at the very least rolled my eyes at his use of the word 'girl'. As it was, I lay there in shamed silence, trying not to dribble, my swollen tongue aching desperately in my mouth.

'You are a silly little girl aren't you?'

Oh no, I thought, please don't do this. Being called a good girl, at a push, is something I felt worrying pangs of joy at by then but this ... I felt myself clamping my lips around the chopsticks and my protruding tongue in silent rebellion.

'Slap my cunt again.'

My first thought was 'whose bloody cunt?' but even as I was forming thoughts of outrage my hand was moving to do his bidding. I thanked him.

'Tell me.'

I sighed. Opened my mouth. Closed it. Tried again. Suddenly the chopsticks seemed to be in the way of my teeth when I tried to speak in the way they weren't a few seconds before.

The shame was audible even if the actual words weren't, thanks to my immobilised tongue. 'I'm a silly little girl.'

'Silly little girls blow raspberries don't they?'

I was whimpering acquiescence to everything he was saying, agreeing desperately to anything that would make this end because it hurt so much and felt so humiliating.

'Can you blow a raspberry now?'

I was gabbling, my words incomprehensible for anything but a lisping tone of desperation. 'No, no I can't.'

'Try,' he hissed.

Come on, Kate, this'll soon be over. This has to be the worst it can get. With tears streaming down my face I tried. Desperately, repeatedly, I blew air out of my mouth, huffing pathetically, my lips unpursed, unpursable desperate for it to end, for my aching jaws to close.

And then of course it got worse.

'Put a hand between your legs. What do you feel?'

I flushed. I knew what I was going to feel as, in spite of everything, I was achingly wet. The increasingly wet sound of the palm of my hand slapping against my cunt had given it away by degrees, even without the glistening proof on my fingers getting stickier with every slap.

'Too shy to say? Press your fingers to that outstretched tongue of yours. Taste yourself. Tell me.'

I moved my hand to my aching mouth and transferred the taste of my body's betrayal of my mind to my throbbing tongue. With gritted teeth I told him what he already knew. 'I'm wet.'

'What?'

In this second I loathed Josh even as I wanted to obey him, to best him with my submission. In my mind this was a competition and I could only win by not wussing out now. Delusional? Possibly. I blame it on the lack of blood to my tongue. Through gritted teeth, I bit out the words: 'My cunt is wet.'

His retort was quick. 'Whose cunt?'

I sighed again, broken, desperate for this to end. 'Your cunt.'

'Good girl.'

At the endearment the loathing dissipated and I felt a burst of pride, before a slight twinge of panic at how conditioned I was becoming.

'Now shove your fingers up inside my cunt and make yourself come. Once I've heard you bring yourself off I will allow you to remove all the clamps.'

I honestly don't know if it would have made it better or worse if I'd come easily at his treatment of me then. For what it's worth, the pain in my tongue and the difficulties I had swallowing away the drool, paired with a deep-felt feeling of humiliation and remorse meant I was distracted and unable to come easily. By the time I begged him for my orgasm, my voice high-pitched and desperate and unintelligible, my body sore and aching, I felt like he had stripped me of everything. I was totally his, for better or worse, and I wouldn't ever make an error like that again.

As I came back to earth, tentatively removing the clamps from my breasts and tongue and feeling the surging agony as blood began pulsing through them again properly, I felt exhausted, utterly spent and oddly upset. I wanted to speak to him, but I didn't know what to say. I felt so ashamed – both at having disappointed him and having just done so many humiliating things at his bidding – that I couldn't shrug the feeling off to converse normally. I felt more tongue-tied than I had with the sodding clamp on.

He was incongruously and yet reassuringly solicitous, asking me if I was OK, whether I needed to find some ice to help with my sore tongue. Ridiculously, his kindness made my eyes fill with tears again.

My voice sounded crackly as I tried to speak, my mouth dry having been forcibly held open for so long. 'I'll be fine, thank you.' I knew I would be, but I also knew this lesson would stay in my mind for a long time, and that I would never look at chopsticks in quite the same way again.

'Good girl.'

I swallowed quietly and with a plaintiveness I couldn't quite shake said, 'I am sorry you know.'

His voice was warm, comforting. 'I know. And if you want I can give you another assignment to make it up to me.'

Even before he'd finished the sentence I was agreeing with him, asking for my chance to make amends. He directed me back to my bag, this time the front outside pocket – I was fast realising I should have paid more attention to what exactly was in my luggage – where there was a small drawstring bag which he told me to pull open. I took out a small vibrator, a buttplug, and a sachet of lube.

As I looked at the collection of items on the edge of my bed my heart started pounding again, not sure after everything that had come before that I could endure anything more that night. He told me he wanted me to plug my own arse, and push the vibrator high into my cunt and write a new assignment, but instead of telling him what I fantasised about us doing when we were reunited he wanted me to explain how I felt during every humiliating moment of the punishment I had just endured, all while stuffed in two holes and desperate to come. I was not to orgasm until I'd finished and emailed the piece to him for him to read and it needed to be at least 2,000 words – unless I came before I'd finished in which case it needed to be an extra 1,000 words for each "accident". And if he didn't have it at some point in the few short hours before I was due to finish up and return home to see him he would punish me again, in person, maybe with the tongue clamp as he knew now how much I hated it and was actually amused at the idea of seeing me try and speak round it while he caned me.

My mouth was dry as I stared with trepidation at the buttplug, which was significantly thicker than anything else I'd had in my arse. My voice wavered. 'It's almost 1 a.m.'

I imagined his smile. 'I know. I should go to bed, I need to get up early for work. I suggest you get started.'

I shoved myself full and, aching all over, sat myself at the little desk in the anonymous hotel room, and wrote, well, most of the words that became this chapter.

Chapter Eleven

BARRING THE EXTENUATING CIRCUMSTANCES of the tongue-clamping debacle, I'd say I'm usually pretty good with deadlines. As a journalist it's drummed into you. You don't miss a deadline. Ever. No ifs, no buts, no maybes. A deadline is a deadline is a deadline. That's it. No matter what pressure you're under or how close to the wire you get, the adrenaline kicks in and you make sure you make it. Because there's no sliding scale. You either hit or you don't. And if you don't then it's game over, whether you've missed the boat by a millimetre or a mile.

But that's when I'm trying to finish a page lead, or put some breaking copy on one of our websites. Sometimes, with the best will in the world, other deadlines seem almost unreachable.

I was crying. Tears had run down my face in rivulets, and splashed onto my naked breasts, tiny drips which did nothing to cool the flush across my chest which signalled both arousal and embarrassment. In a small corner of my mind I was worried there might be a little snot too, but since my hands were handcuffed behind me there was no surreptitious way to brush it away even if that was the case, and suddenly – as he moved – any similarities between me and the woman from the *Blair Witch Project* seemed the least of my worries. His hand tangled viciously in my hair, pulling my head so I was forced to look him in the eye, see his dominance reflected back at my submission.

It was breathtaking, terrifying, and did nothing to help me regain the shattered vestiges of my equilibrium.

My breath was coming fast in little sobs that I was trying my best to swallow, to little avail. I bit my lip, staring past his ear into the middle distance, trying to pull myself together, trying to process the conflicting sensations and emotions flickering through me. Pain. Fear. Excitement.

Josh's voice, so close to me that his breath kissed my face, actually made me jump.

'Do you understand?'

I went to nod, realised that his hand was clamped so tightly into my hair that it would hurt, and instead forced the words through parched and trembling lips.

'Yes, sir.'

Calling him 'sir' was something that came frighteningly easily by then, to the extent I'd even caught myself mentally referring to him that way. He'd made me call him 'Master' a couple of times, although that chafed. That night I would have called him Grand Vizier Smorgasbord of the Planet Zarg if I thought it would help. But it wouldn't. This was a new level of dominance, requiring a new level of submission, and while the pooling of my juice under me proved that I was enjoying stepping up to the plate, I was more on the back foot than ever before.

His voice was charming. 'Good. Well since we've not been counting up to this point, I think we'll assume that I've given you 20 smacks so far. Does that sound reasonable?'

I agreed quickly, eagerly, having no idea how many times he'd hit me but thinking this sounded like a suitably high number. There shouldn't be too much more to endure, I didn't think he'd ever punished me so extensively before so –

'If we count on to a hundred. I think that'll be fair.'

At his words I started trembling again. Harder than I had at any point so far.

It had started with, I thought, a relatively playful pussy spanking. He had me strip and sit on the high-backed chair, spreading my legs wide in the cool seat so he could secure an ankle to each chair leg, leaving me open wide to his gaze – and his hand. He had a definite gleam in his eye when he produced the handcuffs, pulled my hands behind the chair and secured me into place. But it wasn't until he disappeared off to the kitchen and came back with a wooden spoon and two clothes pegs that the alarm bells started ringing fully, and by then there wasn't a huge amount I could do other than struggle ineffectually against the chair. Which it turned out would come later.

He played with my breasts to start with. Running his hands over and around them, his touch soothing, lulling me into a feeling of security. He lightly pinched my nipples, watching them harden, my body basking in his attention. Then he put his mouth around my nipple, lapping at it and suckling deep until I closed my eyes in bliss at the sensation.

I should have known better. Almost as soon as I relaxed into his ministrations, he changed, grazing my nipple with his teeth, his teeth getting harsher, biting until I cried out. My moans of pain didn't stop him though, and both my breasts were wet with his saliva and red with marks from biting and vicious suckling by the time he put the pegs on. My breasts were also sore and, since the pegs were household-style robust wooden clothes pegs, they hurt as the springs snapped back into place making for a whole new layer of agony. I clenched and unclenched my hands in the cuffs, trying to become acclimatised to the pain, blushing at how intently he stared at my breasts, bouncing with the movement of the deep breaths I was pushing through my nose to try and withstand the sensations.

I was so intent on dealing with the tight hot pain in my nipples fast becoming the centre of my world, that I forgot about the spoon until he slapped one of my breasts with it. He'd slapped my breasts with his hands before but this, particularly after the biting and suckling which made my tits look properly tortured, really hurt. The layers of pain were running one on top of another, like conflicting currents, waves rushing in my head. In that moment my entire world was focused only on that noise – and the pain in my nipples.

Up until the point he smacked me hard between the legs with the wooden spoon.

I screamed. I couldn't stop myself. I've never felt pain like it. The silence after my voice pierced the room felt as loud as actual noise. Everything was still, my eyes were filled with tears and it was all silent for a moment bar the sound of my rasping breathing. He didn't ask me if I was all right. He just looked at me very intently, staring into my eyes, while I – undoubtedly – glared back at him, my mind furious at not only him for inflicting this agony but on the part of myself that actually, despite it all, craved it. After a few seconds he must have seen what he needed to see, as then the air changed and he moved.

As he shifted closer I closed my eyes, unable to bear watching a second strike. Of course all that meant – stupidly – was that I wasn't ready for it. The sound of spoon hitting my cunt so directly echoed about the room and the pain felt like nothing I'd ever felt before. In the back of my mind a panicked voice was whimpering "I can't take this" but before I could do anything to stop it (or stop him even – I was closer to doing that than I had ever been before) the third crack connected and I was gasping through the pain and my tears again. Every fibre of my being was focused on the man in front of me and trying to ride the waves of pain he was thwapping into my cunt.

I don't know if it's just me, but normally after a few strokes of whatever implement I am on the receiving end of my body can start to adjust to the pain, embrace it. It still hurts, of course it does, but something alters in my head and the pain starts to bring with it a delicious pleasure. But as he kept up the relentless spanking rhythm of the wooden spoon it only hurt, and then hurt more. I shifted against my bound ankles, desperate to close my legs against the onslaught but unable to do so. All I could do was endure, cling on and hope it would get better, that it wouldn't be the thing I couldn't cope with, that I would have to call a halt, disappointing him and myself. I really wasn't sure I could get through it. Even endure it, never mind enjoying it. But he had different opinions.

That's when he set me my deadline.

He tucked a strand of hair back behind my ear as he explained what would happen next. And it made the world shift for a second as I tried to understand what he was saying. What he was expecting.

'The thing is, even while you're crying and whimpering and shaking this is making you wet.'

I opened my mouth to argue, but before I could speak he pressed the curved end of the spoon against my lips. I tasted myself on the wood, blushed and closed my eyes, to hide the truth in my gaze at my body's betrayal. As he moved the spoon away I pressed my trembling lips together and swallowed the denial, deciding discretion was the better part of valour and I should probably just shut up.

'I think if I spanked you for long enough you could come from me hitting your greedy cunt.'

My eyes flashed open and I looked at him smiling down at me, a picture of smugness. The more we'd played the better he'd got to know my limits. This was sometimes amazing, as when he was pushing me into the unknown it felt like I was flying. However, at other points – points like this when he was looking arrogant as he merrily pushed me into the abyss – I could have quite happily told him to go and fuck himself. Except, as ever, the small voice in my head already yearning for the next time this would happen kept me quiet. For a while.

'So I'm going to give you a deadline. A certain number of strokes by which time you have to come. If you don't, I am going to do things to you that will make this feel like a walk in the park. And if you don't come, well it won't matter to me. Because I will, either by having you suck me off or just giving you a damn good fucking' – at that he ran a hand along my cunt lips which made me buck underneath him as much as I could within the constraints of my bonds – 'and then I will punish you in ways you can't even begin to imagine. You will be begging me and you won't know whether you're begging me to stop or continue. But I will use you however I want, for however long I want until you want to just crawl away and recover. And since neither of us has to be back at work until after the weekend now that could be a very long time. Do you understand?'

I felt fear in the pit of my stomach, excitement, and – ridiculously – the kind of burst of adrenaline that I always get when given something to work to. Yes, I am a journalistic cliché. I was already aching to come and competitive enough that I was going to try and get through this no matter what. I could do this. The pain couldn't go on too long. My voice was quiet but, I like to think, fairly assured. 'Yes, sir.'

'Good. Well since we've not been counting up to this point, I think we'll assume that I've given you 20 smacks so far. Does that sound reasonable? If we count on to a hundred. I think that'll be fair.'

The rhythm was what got me. Even with the pain – and believe me, it was a kind of agony I had never felt before – the insidious rhythm of his strikes against my poor pussy began to work its warmth through me. He made me count off the strokes and thank him for them and his pace was so fast that I was gasping out my thanks as fast as I could speak, as fast as I could process the pain. At stroke 63 the sensations shifted. He hit me, as hard as he had up to that point, but the noise of the wood connecting to my cunt was squelchy. Wet. The sound of my arousal was obvious. And with every hit it got more so, until I closed my eyes in embarrassment. My tears of pain were still streaming from beneath my closed lids, and yet the increasing wet patch I was squirming in, that was coating the back of my thighs and my arse, proved how despite my brain telling me otherwise on a cellular level this was working for me.

At stoke 69 I opened my eyes, and saw him pulling away from the stroke I was still gasping at. My cunt juice was a strand of wetness leading from my pussy to the spoon as he moved away and the visible evidence of how much this pain was turning me on shocked me for a second, freezing my brain. When he hit me again I couldn't think of the number. Were we on 69 and this was 70? Or was this 69? Shit. I guessed, '69.' He shook his head in displeasure and told me we'd go back to 60 to make up for my error. I had to bite my lip to stop myself beginning to sob at the thought of nine extra strokes.

By the time we get to 85 he had shifted the angle he was hitting me at so every strike had maximum impact on my clit. It was the most intense treatment it had ever received and my body was already building up to an orgasm which I feared the strength of. As we moved inexorably closer to 100 my breathing was ragged, my still-pegged nipples jiggling as I gasped and my thighs trembled as I built to my climax.

On the hundredth strike I orgasmed. I would have been rolling my eyes at the fact I had metamorphosed into some ridiculous cliché of slutty kinky conditioning, but, having endured all I'd endured, after every ounce of feeling had been wrung from my body, I didn't give a toss. I wanted to come so much it consumed me. It was all I could taste, all I could smell and I felt like I needed it more than I needed to breathe.

My orgasm was vicious and painful and made me thrash against my bonds in a way that left me with marks round my wrists and ankles that I had to hide with long sleeves and trousers for a few days. The keening noises coming from the back of my throat didn't sound like me and as I came, pulsating around the spoon, Josh had to grab the back of the chair as I was about to tip both it and myself over with the force of my movements.

As I came back down to earth as if coming out of a trance, still shivering with aftershocks from the intensity of what had come before, he was undoing his trousers, pulling his cock out and moving over to me. He pushed his cock viciously inside me, putting his weight onto my still pulsating, puffy, bruised and aching cunt. I couldn't hold back a scream. He started to fuck me, a cruel reminder of the rhythm of the spoon just minutes before, the sensations so painful and intense that I was bucking from underneath him, doing everything I could to push him off which, because of the handcuffs and rope securing my ankles, was very little.

He shifted deeper inside me and then stopped moving for a moment. He anchored his hands in my hair, and kissed me deeply, then bit hard on my bottom lip until I was sure I could taste blood. His fingers twisted on the pegs on my nipples, adjusting and tightening them until it felt like my entire body was on fire. I was sobbing, tears streaming down my face, and as he resumed fucking me he whispered, 'You came on stroke 109 because we went back when you miscounted. You missed your deadline.'

Through a haze of pain and intense pleasure I realised exactly what this meant. And I trembled, knowing over the next minutes, hours, days, however long he wanted, I was going to be pushed further than I ever had been before.

No ifs, no buts, no maybes. You never miss a deadline.

The days that followed were the most challenging of my life. He used me. Abused me. Humiliated me. Slapped me with his cock. Spat in my face. Put pegs on my cunt lips. He made me cry. He made me ache. He challenged me. Pushed me. He never broke me but at times it felt like he was trying. He fucked me, when he wanted, how he wanted, and when I was so exhausted I could not summon up the energy to do anything more than lie there, a fuckhole for his pleasure, he slapped my face and pulled my hair to make me move my weary body. By the time he finished I was marked all over, like an abstract canvas documenting our time together. The bite marks on my breasts, the angry redness of my tormented nipples. The bruises on the tops of my arms, the slashes of the red welts criss-crossing both arse cheeks that made me squirm, made me wet thinking of what had happened for weeks afterwards. His spunk drying in my hair and on my tits. By the end the tracks of my tears had washed away carefully applied make up, my hair was a mess, I was a mess. He had demolished my defences.

It was freeing, cathartic and yet at points terrifying. He pushed me to the very edge of what felt acceptable to me. As the hours and days passed all I cared about was him – pleasing him, satisfying him, not doing anything to give him reason to punish me. He was my world and for the first time I truly understood the kind of submission which consumes you as, for the first time ever, the voice in the back of my head, calling out my shame, asking me why I was doing this, was silenced. I felt connected to him in a way that I never had to another person – he understood me completely, even when I didn't understand myself. As I sobbed, begging him to stop caning me, pleading that I couldn't take any more and he continued anyway I hated him. But he pulled my face to his, his hands hard on my chin and, while I stared at him with loathing in my eyes, he asked me if I remembered my safeword. Through gritted teeth I said yes, and while I battled with stubborn pride and a competitive spirit that meant I then lapsed into silence, he made me beg him to resume before he started again. He caned me until it hurt so much I couldn't breathe, until I was sure I must be bleeding, and then, when he felt I couldn't take any more, he ran a leisurely finger down my slit. I came, from this gentlest of touches, and when I came back to earth, sated and yet confused at how the caning could have inspired such a vicious orgasm, I saw him smiling down at me, leaning to kiss me softly before he told me I would have to be punished for coming without permission.

When he finally finished he tethered me to the foot of the bed like an animal, my wrists tied behind my back, and left me to sleep the sleep of the exhausted, curled in an ungainly way, unconsciously trying to find a part of my body to lie on comfortably.

It may sound odd that such cruelty and humiliation inspired the thought, but by the end of our weekend I knew I loved this twisted, clever, tender man who got upset at people being cruel to animals but took joy in doing horrible things to me that made my head spin. It was the most intense experience of my life.

Chapter Twelve

So what happens after the most intense sexual experience of your life, the thing that leaves you aching and mentally and physically affected for days afterwards?

Well, it would seem, the answer was nothing.

When we said goodbye he was quiet but no more so than he would normally have been at the prospect of us going back to our respective homes, the weekend over and work beginning again. At least that's what I thought at the time, when I stretched up to kiss him, enjoying the warmth of his embrace as he hugged me goodbye and we went our separate ways.

I texted him when I got home, the way I always did. I didn't get a reply but figured that as it was late he'd crashed out in readiness for his early start the next day. But the next morning I didn't hear anything, in fact at no point through the day. It was odd – Josh and I had spent months in contact multiple times a day and his silence meant I couldn't help but worry that something was wrong. I sent him a second text just asking him all was OK. Nothing. Then I tried dropping him an email – a link to a news story I thought might interest him – I didn't want to seem clingy, although I sent it to both his home and work addresses, but I wanted a response, probably dropping into conversation the fact he'd lost his phone.

Nothing.

For three days I was pretty much beside myself. Texts and an aiming-for-casual-and-bright-but-really-not voicemail went unanswered. I went about my daily business, going to work, heading out for birthday drinks with a friend, but through it all in the back of my mind all I was thinking about was Josh. Was he all right? Why hadn't he got in touch? On the morning of the fourth day I couldn't stand it any more. I rang his office. I didn't give my name, which perhaps makes me sound less like a mad stalker woman. The receptionist was very helpful, yes he was definitely in, she'd seen him this morning, he was at his desk already, but on another call. Did I want to leave a message or did I have his address to email him?

I told her I had his address and very politely hung up.

I was furious. I was upset. I was confused. It was so unlike him, but I couldn't really think of the best way to deal with it at that given moment – short of knowing that any kind of attempt at talking to him while he was at work was a complete waste of time – so I spent most of the day thinking about the best way to raise my concerns without seeming like some furious harridan. There was also the D/s dynamic to factor into it. After the intensity of the time we had spent together I didn't want to come across as disrespectful, although that said, I had no intention whatsoever of letting it go like some kind of wilting flower. But what to do?

By the end of the working day I still had no clue.

I decided to send a casual, non-shrewish, text.

Hey you, you've been really quiet since we got back from the weekend. Hope all's OK, will try ringing tonight.

I didn't get a reply. In my heart of hearts I wasn't expecting one, although I still had no fucking clue why.

The cliché of the break-up is that once you have been

spurned by your beau you sink into the pit of despair with some high-quality ice cream and cheesy pop rock of the 70s and early 80s. If that works for you then great. But for me, to paraphrase Billy Ocean, when the going gets tough, the tough get baking.

I rang Josh twice that night and it went to voicemail both times. Then I switched on my PC and, thanks to the joys of social networking, found that he'd been online in various places that evening, happy to talk even if he apparently didn't have the inclination to do so with me. By the time I'd hunted down a post he'd made to an obscure music website asking for help with his speakers – I'm lying here with an aching heart and and a pounding head wondering what on earth's going on and you're recabling your living room? – I knew it was time to step away and do something else.

I'm not a natural cook. Living alone makes anything other than ready meals a lot of hassle and waste for something that I'm usually bored with the prospect of eating part way through the cooking process. But baking, baking I love. Partly I guess because biscuits and cakes and all that stuff are good comfort-type foods, but partly because I enjoy the straightforwardness of it. If you weigh the ingredients out correctly, if you cream the butter and sugar to the right consistency, if you bake it the right length of time you can create something lovely – and you can give the fruits of your efforts to the people around you in silent apology for walking around permanently close to tears and with a face like a smacked arse.

It was 1 a.m. when I decided to start baking ginger shortbread. I don't know why ginger appealed specifically, but I was convinced. By this point I had already drunk most of a bottle of wine, so driving wasn't an option. I pulled my coat on and walked to the 24-hour petrol station with attached shop to buy what I needed there.

Now I've never been the sort of person who buys petrol – or indeed anything else – at a petrol station forecourt late at night. But it turns out that they lock the doors and instead serve you through a glass window with a grill, not unlike visiting someone in prison, passing things underneath the – very small – gap in the bottom of the plexiglass screen.

This made explaining the needs of my late-night baking rather more complicated than it would have been otherwise.

To start with the bloke behind the counter was adamant that unless I wanted fuel, cigarettes or condoms he couldn't sell me anything else. After listening to me argue for five minutes he grudgingly told me he thought they had some flour he could get me. Once he'd cracked and got that it didn't take much wheedling to get some sugar out of him, although by the time I was asking him to hold up packs of butter to see if I could ascertain which was unsalted there was a look of loathing in his eyes. He gave me short shrift when I asked if they had any ginger – admittedly it was unlikely, but clearly heartbreak and drunkenness hadn't dented my optimistic streak – and instead sold me a bar of fruit and nut chocolate to break up in lieu of chocolate chips. By the time I had fed the cash for my overpriced grocery shopping under the gap and he had passed through a carrier bag and then each individual item for me to pack into it, I was so effusively grateful that my eyes were filled with tears at his kindness. As I stumbled away home I think his probably were too – albeit of relief that the mental woman buying baking ingredients had sodded off to leave him with late-night petrol buyers and stoners with the munchies.

I woke up the next morning on my living room floor having passed out watching DVDs while waiting for the second load of shortbread dough to chill in the fridge ready for baking.

If it seems tough waking up with a hangover having been dumped (apparently, it's hard to tell when the person you're dating – well almost – is such an emotional fucktard that you're not entirely sure), then waking up in a furnace – the oven had been on all night, obviously – to find a kitchen in carnage is worse. There was flour on the floor, butter on the cupboards from my overenthusiastic greasing, and every bowl and wooden spoon I owned seemed to have been used and dumped on the side. It was like I'd been burgled. By bakers. Combine that with a banging red wine hangover, sleep deprivation and – as I found when I dragged my sorry self up to the shower – dough in my hair, I felt awful.

I went into work, still not really there, although the batches of shortbread did much to minimise any co-worker snarking about me not pulling my weight. And I tried not to think about Josh. Although thinking about not thinking about Josh didn't count. Probably.

In the weeks that followed my colleagues, friends and family did well out of my heartbreak. I made endless variations of golden shortbread, only moving onto Victoria sponges when our assistant editor raised concerns about all the butter having an effect on his cholesterol. I made carrot cake, rock cakes, cookies, and as I beat the eggs, stirred the dough and waited for everything to cook I went over every element of my relationship with Josh, the smutty and the not so smutty. It made me cry and it made me wet and more than anything it made me angry. I couldn't work out whether everything that happened had been founded on the lie that he was as interested in me as I was in him, if he had got bored with me or I'd done something to piss him off or what, but however I weighed it up, he had thrown away something that from my end seemed quite special. Thrown me away. And it sounded pathetic, made me feel pathetic, but I was bereft and I wanted to weep. Josh still hadn't got in touch, although a mixture of stubborn pride and embarrassment made me stop contacting him. I knew he was alive and well, and over and above that all I knew was that he didn't want to talk to me. And that meant I didn't want to talk to him. I'd be buggered before he realised how much he'd hurt me.

I was part way through grating cheese for a batch of three-cheese scones when Russell rang. He asked how I was. I said I was fine as I was long since bored with trying to explain the ridiculous depth of my feeling to anyone else. And then he shocked me out of slicing lumps off a truckle of Wensleydale.

'Bollocks are you fine. You're not fine.'

I didn't know what to say for a second at the fury and frustration of his tone. I went to say I was fine – by this point it really was my default response – and tailed off as, it would appear, we both knew I wasn't.

'It's enough moping, Kate. More than enough. I'm sorry you're hurting and he's a fucking idiot but no more crying and no more bloody baking. You're coming out with Sarah and me this weekend. No arguments.' He named a fetish club that we'd been talking about going to for ages. 'Get dressed up and we'll pick you up at nine. I'm going to bring the paddle and if you don't cheer up then I will use it.'

I smiled my first unforced smile for weeks. 'Bloody hell, I'd best make an effort then.'

I'd never been to a fetish club before. Don't get me wrong, I was tempted but, as someone a bit self-conscious when dressed up, going somewhere populated by a load of people preening and showing off the shininess of their PVC didn't appeal. Russell had been to a couple and, having realised I was curious and a bit tempted to try, had been extolling the virtues of a couple of different clubs in the city for a few months.

'They aren't like typical London clubs, Kate. They're not posh and filled with people more concerned about what they're wearing than what they're doing. But at the same time, it's not like that club I went to in Manchester.'

The club Russ went to in Manchester had become the stuff of legend. He had gone primarily hoping to play with a girl he'd been chatting to for a while. As he explained to anyone who'd listen, multiple times, with the story becoming more elaborate with each telling, he'd found a lot of tubby people in leather, a bit of shagging, a lot of pretentious D/s posturing that made him bite the inside of his cheek to avoid laughing and a finger buffet. With sausages on sticks.

So yes, he'd earmarked a night out. With some burlesque – which was always going to get my vote – some play space, a couple of potential interesting workshops and not too much wanky posturing. Allegedly.

Of course despite worrying about the flashy clothes horses, my first thought was what to wear. After much thought I chose a low-cut top I usually left in the wardrobe as being a bit too revealing and a skirt short enough that, once I'd put some stockings and a suspender belt underneath it and a pair of chunky heels on my feet, made me feel sexy and yet not too on show. While Russell's threat about the paddle was in the forefront of my mind, I was fairly sure he was joking, but I still chose my favourite midnight blue satin bra and knickers set to go underneath. I had no idea what was going to happen, but hell, going out in good underwear is always to be commended, right?

When Sarah and Russell arrived at my door my jaw dropped open. Sarah had spiked up her short hair with gel and gone heavier than usual on her make-up and looked stunning. Russell meanwhile was wearing a black roll-neck jumper, leather trousers and big boots, and waved the paddle at me with a grin. Between them they looked like a striking pair and for a second I felt a little pang of loneliness at their obvious coupleyness.

Well I did until Sarah pushed her way past me into my flat and, as I turned round, grabbed the back of my head to pull my mouth in for a kiss. For a split second I struggled in confusion, before the taste of her on my mouth and her hands on my arse, tracing over the lines of my skirt to feel for the edge of my knickers, began to arouse me. As my nipples hardened in my bra I sighed softly into her mouth and as I opened in surrender her tongue flickered softly, drawing me deeper.

When she stepped back we were both breathing hard and Russell, who had been standing nearby watching intently, had a prominent erection.

She tucked a stray strand of hair behind my ear. 'Welcome back little girl. Now, shall we go and have some fun?'

For the first time in weeks I was excited at the prospect of what the evening could bring. Josh bloody who? I leant down to pick up my handbag from the sofa. 'Let's go.'

The club was busy by the time we arrived. Russell was right, it wasn't too intimidating walking through the doors, although I was definitely one of the more casually dressed people there. The club itself was an odd and intriguing mixture of the familiar and the unknown. The thumping beats and dark corners of the dance floor in the main room reminded me of a nightclub I frequented often while at uni, down even to the slightly sticky floor from one too many spilled drinks. But the seating dotted around the edge of the main room, plush sofas and banquettes, housed men and women who didn't look like the average bunch of freshers.

There was a lot of leather, PVC and vinyl, as you'd expect, although the sight that made my throat dry and my breath catch was a stunning woman a little shorter than me in a black latex outfit so tight that she may as well have been completely naked. She walked past as we arrived and much to both Russell's and Sarah's amusement I couldn't stop my head turning to get a good look at her arse as she walked past.

Sarah smiled. 'Careful, your shameless lechery is getting to Russellish proportions.'

I rolled my eyes in mock horror – Russell, for all his smooth moves and sexiness, had a reputation for being rather incapable of hiding his facial expressions of admiration after a few drinks. 'Really, that bad? Oh dear.'

Sarah put her hand in mine. 'I think it's a good thing actually.' I looked bemused. 'No, not the leching but the fact you're looking again. It's better than scouring recipe books for new things to do with flour isn't it?'

I blushed. 'I didn't see you complaining when I brought over that lemon drizzle cake.'

She kissed my hand. 'I wasn't complaining. It's just nice to see you showing an interest in anyone again. It looked like you'd taken a battering for a while there.'

I thought back to the various phone calls from both

Russell and Sarah inviting me over for everything from cathartic, mind-blowing sex to watching DVDs, eating takeaway and dissecting Josh's many character faults, and the plethora of increasingly lame excuses I had used to avoid seeing them.

'I'm sorry. I just didn't want to see anyone or do anything. It's not you. Not either of you. I just…' I tailed off. 'I just wasn't in the mood.' After a moment's pause I thought I'd best clarify. 'Either kind of mood.'

Sarah nodded. 'We got that. To be honest, the way you sounded on the phone, I was convinced you were going to take a vow of celibacy and become a nun. If I was a betting woman I'd say you weren't even wanking.'

My jaw dropped open and I looked around desperately to see if anyone had overheard. 'Sarah!'

She smiled and moved closer. 'Don't worry, little one, nobody can hear.' She pressed a soft kiss to one of my flushed cheeks. 'And anyway, it's not as if I've not seen you do lots of filthy things way more depraved than a bit of wanking is it?'

Dammit, she was right. On both counts.

After a couple of hours, and a glass of surprisingly good wine, I was feeling a little more in my element. While I wasn't wandering around on a leash or anything – not a blimmin' chance – people seemed to pick up on the dynamic between Sarah, Russell and I, meaning any approaches came to Russ first and there was none of the lame chat-ups or awkwardness of a normal club as people started getting drunk.

Of course that wasn't the only difference. Apart from the girl I had mentally labelled "lovely latex lady" and the other stunning outfits, there was a fantastic burlesque performance and various rooms round the outside with things going on that pricked my curiosity, even if I wasn't sure if I was brave enough to actually peek round the door and see what was happening.

Sarah had gone to chat with a friend she hadn't seen for a while when Russell – as restless and incapable of sitting still as ever – clambered to his feet. 'Come on, let's go take a look down the rabbit hole shall we? I know you're intrigued to see. Plus, I think they're running a couple of short workshop things that could be fun.'

I followed him.

The first room was bigger than I expected, fairly dark and dotted with half a dozen people being punished and a few more watching them. We stood at the edge of the room, not invading anyone else's space, but listening to the sounds of slaps, smacks and strokes and then the little gasps and whimpers of the people receiving them.

A girl bent over a table with her skirt up caught my attention. I took a couple of steps towards her, before suddenly realising I wasn't sure about the etiquette of it. Her dom caught my eye and nodded slightly, so I took that as an OK to keep watching, although I stepped back a little, feeling Russell move in behind me.

Watching someone else being punished was a slightly surreal experience. Having been on the receiving end of the cane often myself I could imagine intensely how she felt as it kept coming down, and couldn't restrain a shudder at a couple of the swishes which caught her in a way that made her cry out in agony. I felt a pang for her when her dom stopped for a moment and a flash of hope that it was over filled her tear-streaked face, only for it to disappear as he squeezed her arse until she whimpered and then began caning her again. Seeing her facial expressions, and those of her dom, was really arousing and feeling Russ's erection growing against my arse as he stood behind me made me think it wasn't just me feeling that way. It did make me wonder exactly what I looked like in the moment, dealing with the pain, and suddenly I had an insight into why Russell had enjoyed watching me submit to Sarah quite so much – and an urge to see Sarah submit to Russell in similar fashion. I wondered if I could get him to make her hump his leg.

After a few minutes of watching the relentless caning the sub was taking – honestly, I don't think it's something I'd have been able to manage – Russell led me by the arm on to the next room. I glanced over my shoulder at the mess of angry stripes on her arse as we walked past, making me wince in sympathy, even while my nipples hardened in excitement at it. I felt a pang at going, but didn't demur. And then walking through the next door made my jaw drop.

I've always been a bit curious about rope. Obviously, back in the day, my Maid Marion fantasies often involved being tied up but, let's face it, unless you're a camper or own a boat or something there's not really any reason for you to have rope kicking around your house to experiment with. Since I'd started playing in D/s terms I'd been restrained in various ways – with Josh particularly fond of a set of wide leather cuffs for wrists and ankles which could be fastened together with or without chains in a variety of ways to leave me immobile and on display.

But rope? I'd never really seen anyone using rope up close before.

We walked into what seemed to be the end of a workshop on what I assumed was shibari. Whatever it was it looked pretty and the sight of a woman bound with an intricate looping of ropes around her arms and torso, tied at shoulder blade, elbow, wrist and then waist made my throat go a little dry. As I stood staring at her and wondering what it felt like to be tied in that way, Russell huffed slightly under his breath beside me.

I think it was safe to say that Russell didn't really see the appeal of rope.

We watched as the guy giving the demonstration finished his spiel and a ripple of applause signified the end of his workshop. As people started to disappear to get drinks or head into other rooms I moved closer to look at the bound woman. The first thing that struck me was how striking the soft white rope looked against her body – this wasn't the kind of hairy boat-mooring stuff, it was silky and contrasted with her tanned, soft skin in a way that made me want to stroke both her and the rope. Although in my fantasies Maid Marion was never topless.

I looked up to see her watching me, and I blushed, aware I was treating her somewhat like a piece of meat. OK, she probably didn't mind, you'd assume modelling for this kind of thing it was par for the course, but even so. I felt I'd best say something.

'Does it hurt?'

She smiled at me. 'No, not at all. I need to be fairly limber sometimes depending on the position Mark puts me in before he starts,' she grinned. 'It's OK though, I do yoga.'

Never one to miss out on the chance to talk to a topless woman, Russell had moved towards us. He just about managed to hide the sneer from his voice as he spoke, although the bafflement was audible. 'Don't you find it boring? Spending hours having rope wound and rewound around your body while you just stand or kneel or whatever?'

She opened her mouth to speak, but was interrupted by, I don't know, her partner, colleague, wrangler

191

technically I suppose, the guy running the workshop. He'd finished selling rope and books to audience members from a table in the corner and come over to see what was going on. 'It's not boring, either for the person doing the ropework or the person being tied, and it doesn't take hours.'

Russell rolled his eyes. 'Oh come on. It's all very well showing it to people here in a half-hour slot, but let's face it a scout's badge for knotting skills and some patience isn't going to get you very far. Something like that must take hours to learn, and hours more of practice.'

Ropeman just laughed. 'It's dead easy. With a couple of ten-metre lengths of rope and a bit of guidance you could do something in twenty minutes here now.' He wandered towards the table. 'And I have the rope.'

For all that Russell goes on about me being stubborn and bloody-minded, in the right mood he is even worse. And the glint in his eyes was such that I knew exactly where this was going, and that we wouldn't be leaving this room for a little while. He threw open his arms. 'OK then, show me.' He looked at his watch. 'I bet it takes more than twenty minutes though.'

Pretty much exactly twenty minutes later I was topless too, my breasts bound with the same kind of soft rope. Now don't get me wrong, I hadn't really come out that night intending to end up with my bra off and my baps out, but when Ropeman – who by this point we were just calling Mark – suggested breast binding it was a natural progression. We were tucked away in a side room after all and, barring the odd person sticking their head round the door, it was fairly secluded.

Mark started by looping a long piece of rope folded double around my waist under my breasts. Then he

192

wound it round and round, firmly and neatly with each pass sitting flat next to the previous one, then tying off the end in the small of my back. Taking a second long loop of rope he had Russell do the same, this time just above the curve of my breasts, but in exactly the same way. It took a little longer than Mark's first pass, mainly because at one point the rope got crossed, and Russell had to unloop it and try again. By the time he'd tied off his piece of rope, though, my breathing was already feeling surprisingly constricted and my breasts were swelling through the rope as the feeling of increased restraint aroused me.

The third piece of rope is where what they were doing started to look more like artistry. Russell looped it under both of the first two lots at my breast bone and pulled tightly, so suddenly the circlets round my body met, tightening round into a diamond between my breasts. Then the looping began. Round and round and round each individual breast in a figure of eight, tight and neat and unyielding. As the amount of turns increased my breasts began to look more distended in their bondage and my breath caught at how beautiful it looked.

My nipples were hard and tight, not only because of the excitement of being tied, but also oddly because of the treatment I was getting at Mark and Russell's hands. The impersonal way they moved my breasts, put a hand on my shoulder, began to make me feel really wet. The fact they weren't touching me in a way that was at all sexual just seemed to make it more arousing, and I found that after a while I was drifting off, not listening to Mark explaining to Russell exactly how he should be twisting the rope, or how to make sure he was keeping things tight but not too tight, and instead standing compliant while they worked. It was liberating and surprisingly soothing, a chance to let my mind wander.

Once the final piece of rope had been tied off, Mark began explaining to Russell how to bind me effectively at the elbow and wrist in a way that wouldn't cut off circulation and which would, apparently, push my breasts out even further. After a second's pause so Russell could ask if I minded them giving it a go, tinged with a boyish glee that I imagined was how he used to be playing with Lego, before I knew it my hands were tied behind me.

The whole experience left me wet and a little inarticulate. Surprisingly so, actually. I'd always known rope was something I'd like to try, but hadn't expected it to be so affecting when basically we were being given a bit of sales spiel to get us to buy some rope from a bloke hawking it from a little table like a stall on an indoor market. It was so relaxing. I felt a little outside myself, the way you do after a lovely massage. And as I looked down at my breasts, round and red like pomegranates, full and aching, for the first time in ages I felt free and like I wasn't thinking about Josh.

And then he spoke. 'When you've got a pair of breasts as well secured and lush looking as that, they're just asking for a cropping.'

For a second I thought I'd imagined him, was mentally kicking myself for failing in my 'not thinking about Josh' pledge. But then I looked up and there he was, leaning against the door frame. He looked tired, but irritatingly still sexy enough to make me feel a pang.

Russell moved between us. He'd never met Josh before, had no reason to know what he looked like, and so in his mind was glaring at some dominant making lewd comments about someone he didn't know. Normally I'd have mocked him, asked him if he wanted to piss on me to mark his ownership, but in that moment I'd have hugged him if my hands weren't bound. Instead I stepped round him.

'It's OK.' I thought I'd best try and calm things, and – ever the polite one – nodded my head to make some introductions. 'Russell this is Josh. Josh, Russell.' If anything, knowing who he was made Russell look more likely to do Josh some kind of harm, so I half turned to him. 'Russ, it's fine. Honestly. Although I would like you to untie my arms. Now.'

One look at my face and Russell knew to move into action. He began ineffectually trying to undo the first knot at my wrist, his hands fumbling under the pressure of my fury. My eyes still on Josh, as though if I blinked he'd disappear, I managed to hiss out of the corner of my mouth. 'If you're having trouble just cut me free.'

Mark piped up then. 'Rope's very expensive you know, if you're cutting through it you have to buy it.' Brilliant. Not only was I in some kind of fetish floor show, but it was going to cost me the price of a lovely pair of shoes for the privilege. To his credit, Russell got my arms cut free and stumped up. While he was talking to Mark about what he owed – I heard him squeak 'how much?' – I walked across the room to Josh.

When I reached him he had the decency to look embarrassed. 'Hi. Sorry to interrupt.'

I actually wanted to swing for him, although in the end I crossed my arms over my bound and still-mostly-naked breasts and made do with glaring instead. As a journalist I'm fully aware of the power of silence. I said nothing.

After a few seconds he cracked. 'I didn't think fetish clubs were your kind of place really.'

Yeah, of course you fucking didn't, I thought. Otherwise you wouldn't have risked seeing me here.

I aimed for a carefree shrug. 'I came along with some friends, thought I'd extend my social circle a bit and have some fun.'

He nodded. 'That sounds like a really good idea.'

I nodded back. 'Well yes, it is a way of meeting like-minded people.'

Jesus, who knew you could have a D/s tinged conversation as mindless and bland as discussing the weather? I felt a pang of guilt for emptying Russ's wallet for this.

Suddenly Josh's eyes were staring intently into mine, looking for answers in a way that reminded me so much of how he looked to see whether I could stand any more punishment that my heart hurt. His tone was abrupt. 'Is that what you're doing then? Looking to meet new like-minded people?'

I felt a surge of anger. He'd been lovely and filthy and sexy and mean and once I'd fallen for him he dumped me without telling me why, turning me into a heartbroken baker, and he had the temerity to be hacked off with me? I couldn't stop myself.

'What's it to you?' He flinched at the fury in my voice. 'Seriously. What is it to you, Josh? If there's one thing the last month has made painfully obvious it's that you're not interested in continuing to explore what was happening between us. That's fine. You can't fake a connection, although actually I thought you were emotionally capable enough that if you wanted us to stop seeing each other you'd at least let me know.' A flush formed on his cheeks. 'But do you know what? I don't care. Honestly I don't. You aren't the person I thought you were. I was hoping you were the real deal, someone who complemented me, completed me even, in kinky and vanilla ways. I thought you were that person but then I realised you aren't. And now I don't care. I fell for someone who it turns out didn't actually exist. That's my mistake, for being naïve and taking what you said at face value. I'll learn from that. But don't you dare try and guilt trip me. Don't you dare.'

For a second the room was silent. I never lose my temper like that. I couldn't tell you the last time I did. I could see Russell open-mouthed in my peripheral vision, while Josh's eyes were wide.

He put his hand on my arm. 'Kate, I –'

I pushed him off with such force I shocked myself and almost knocked him over. 'Don't you touch me. We're done.'

And then I stalked out of the room. Afterwards, when he'd found me and given me my bra and top back and undone the breast binding, Russ told me I looked like Xena Warrior Princess's furious and more skimpily dressed sister. By that point the anger had dissipated and I was tearful, embarrassed and drinking a fortifying glass of wine with him and Sarah. Although part of me wished I'd had Xena's sodding sword for the occasion.

Chapter Thirteen

I VERY RARELY LOSE my temper properly. I'm as prone to a rant as the next woman, but generally in life I'm fairly easy-going. My confrontation with Josh was completely out of character, to the extent that both Russell and – once he'd explained the gist of what had happened to her – Sarah were both a little agog.

The rest of the evening passed so inoffensively as to be anti-climactic. I got dressed and Russell collected the remains of his very expensive rope. We found Sarah and had a couple more drinks before watching a burlesque act. Josh seemed to have gone home. I like to think I was carrying off a carefree and light-hearted demeanour, although I caught Sarah and Russ exchanging concerned glances at several points so perhaps I wasn't. But overall, I was doing OK. Getting everything off my chest felt oddly cathartic, and had helped draw a line under everything. And I didn't even feel like making a batch of scones, which had to be progress.

So I got home, had a bit of a cry – when you only lose your temper properly once every couple of years there's an emotional hangover to be had there – and went to bed, feeling at least like I'd got it out of my system. Until I woke up the next morning and checked my phone.

Hey, was good to see you yesterday. Fancy meeting for a trip to the cinema or something? – J xx

I read and reread the text. Two kisses? That suggested something, right? But what? And did I even want to know? Was it worth risking it? What was stopping him from pulling the same stunt a few weeks down the line?

There were two different schools of thought, summed up neatly by Russell and Sarah. Russ thought the best thing I could do was refuse to meet him, draw a line under everything, and start moving on. Sarah thought I should go along, be friendly but unflirty, wear a killer outfit and leave him regretting what he'd given up. After a couple of days of dithering – no more replying to texts within half an hour – I decided to go with the latter strategy. Which, yes, may be proof of my masochistic tendencies.

So I found myself heading over to see a film I wasn't that interested in seeing, wearing an outfit with arguably a little more cleavage showing than I'd normally have been showing on a trip to the flicks. And why? I'm not entirely sure even now. The film was good, the banter between us non-flirty but easy-going enough. And when I popped back to collect my car from parked outside his place and Josh asked me up for a cup of coffee I said yes although, if asked, why I wouldn't have been able to say why.

But it seemed I wasn't the only one not exactly capable of explaining what was going on in my head. He was fiddling about with the coffee machine when he started talking: 'I don't know if you noticed me cooling off quite abruptly.' My mouth gaped open at the understatement. 'And I couldn't have explained it to you, didn't really know what was going on, which sounds stupid, I know. But something has clicked for me this evening. And I didn't even realise it till now.'

And then he told me. He told I was amazing and that intellectually he thought I was one of the most intelligent, interesting people he'd met for ages, that I made him laugh, that he really enjoyed spending time with me – all lovely things I've mentally filed away for retrieval during those crap days where I feel rubbish about myself. But then, as my inner monologue was gearing itself up for the "but" that explained why despite all this good stuff he'd hotfooted it away like the hounds of hell were after him, he told me something that made me look up, confused, thinking I'd misheard him.

'The more I like you, the more time we spend together, the harder it is for me to dominate you, Kate. To hurt you. When we first played, seeing the apprehension in your eyes, hearing you whimper, made me hard. But now, it's upsetting. And I'm sorry.'

What do you say in that situation? Well I said very little, in part because if I'd sat down and wrote a list of possible reasons for what had happened between us, this wouldn't have been in the first hundred. And as he kept talking, and apologised, over and over again, so embarrassed you'd think he was admitting he was suffering from premature ejaculation, my first instinct was to give him a hug, and tell him everything would be all right.

We were silent for a little while, before my brain finally kicked in enough to ask why it hadn't been a problem before.

Running a hand through his hair he told me he'd never dominated anyone in person as violently as he had me. That he respected me more than anyone he'd played with previously in the sense that I was more capable, more equal to him, and while on an academic level dominating me turned him on, hence him talking a good game via email, in person he increasingly found it difficult whether I was glowering up at him or had my eyes filled with tears. And then he apologised some more. Lots more. To the point where I did just give him a big hug, and we drank our coffee.

He'd been staring into his mug for a little while before I finally got my thoughts in order enough to speak, not even sure whether it would or should make a difference, but feeling more than ever that the final piece of the puzzle had dropped into place, and that maybe – actually – Josh needed to hear it too, even if it was difficult for me to say.

'When you hurt me I like it. I crave it even. I don't know whether you can tell that when I'm glaring at you, when my eyes are filled with tears, when I'm blushing, even when I can't quite hide my expression of fear at the thought of whatever fiendish thing you're going to do next. Being so completely on the back foot, being demeaned, being hurt, diminished, does it for me. Feeling your hands at my wrists, at my throat, or in my hair, feeling you overpower me, master me, makes my breath quicken. It makes me wet. I lie in bed at night thinking about it sometimes.'

I took a big gulp of coffee – this was way harder than admitting I was a slut or begging for orgasm and, somehow, felt like one of the most important conversations of my life, no matter what happened. I continued, peeking over my mug to see his reaction.

'Yes, you hurt me. But you do it with my permission. I beg you to do it, literally sometimes. Hurting me isn't a bad thing in this context. The fact that you're you – kind, intelligent, polite, lovely Josh – is what makes me feel confident and safe enough for you to do that. I wouldn't give any old person the power over me that I give you. In fact I've never given any other person the extent of the power over me that I've given you, not even Russell. And I give you this power *because* of the vanilla you. If you were as merciless and harsh all the time as you are when you're choking me then I wouldn't want to play with you.

'Don't get me wrong, when you're doing that, when you're cocking an eyebrow at me, when you're making me whimper, it's hot enough to make my nipples harden and my cunt wet just thinking about it. But I like the paradox. I like both sides of you. I like the fact I can trust you to hurt me, to take pleasure in having the power to make me cry, and yet still be thoughtful and lovely enough afterwards to give me a hug, make sure that I'm physically and mentally OK, get me a glass of wine or some juice. That is a good thing. These two sides of you aren't contrary to each other. They fit together perfectly, and both show a considerateness and awareness of other people's needs. Hurting someone who wants to be hurt is not only not a bad thing, it's practically a cathartic kindness.'

He was sitting completely still. I put my hand on his arm, trying to make him understand, fearing that actually my words weren't going to be enough, which all things considered is pretty bloody ironic.

'As I said, I'm hoping you know this already. And don't worry, I'm not telling you this because I'm trying to wangle my way into a relationship with you.' I suddenly realised I was sounding aloof by accident and tried to clarify. 'Don't get me wrong, I'm not saying I wouldn't be interested in trying one – it's not every day I get to meet someone as lovely, intelligent, challenging, sexy and twisted as you. I have so much fun and enjoy being with you in and out of bed. But I don't know that you're in the right place for a relationship now even if you were interested in pursuing one with me specifically – and I'm not assuming that either. But if nothing else happens between us except us exchanging moans via email and meeting for an occasional beer I think you need to hear this anyway.'

I put my mug down. 'Yes, you're sadistic. And maybe you need to get your head round that, to figure out whether you're happy being that person. But for me, I'm happy with you being both the man my mum would want me to bring home and the one she'd warn me about in one complex, interesting, fascinating package. And I'm happy being me – needing to be hurt, craving it, wanting to be humiliated and demeaned, loving being challenged and being pushed and sometimes pushing back.'

We sat in silence for a little while. When it became apparent he wasn't ready to speak yet I decided it was time to brave the traffic home. I picked my handbag from the floor and my coat from the back of the chair. 'If you figure out that you're happy in the same way, then give me a call.'

And then I left. Because suddenly it all made sense, even in the context of the fucked-up, messy emotions of whatever was happening with Josh and me. If he was my soulmate, the person I was to end up with, my dom, my partner, then it would happen from this. And if he didn't, well I'd been honest, and I knew what I was looking for now.

And I knew it was worth waiting for.

Epilogue

IT'S BEEN ONE OF those weeks.

One of those weeks where I haven't been able to switch off, where the trials and tribulations of day-to-day life have been so overarching that sex has been the last thing on my mind and just getting through without my brain imploding has felt like a real stretch. Juggling long, busy and stressful work days with evenings spent writing to finish this book in time for my deadline. Thinking more about my nature – submissive and otherwise – than I ever have before and trying to put it into words that are both sexy and truthful, even when sometimes the self-awareness that comes out of that brings me up short. Ironically, all this has meant my orgasms have been grabbed purely to bring on the blessed relief of sleep, the very definition of 'all work and no play'.

So when I come into the room and see him sitting at my PC, leisurely stroking his cock while reading through a chapter I'd cast aside a few days before, I didn't see it as a prelude to an afternoon of shagging.

But as every sub knows, often it's not down to you.

Getting into the sub mindset comes easier some times than others. And right now, with my head filled with the myriad of shit that's been going on for the last week or so, I'm light years away from any kind of obedient submissive best – and let's face it, I have a problem with the obedient at the best of times. If only he didn't look so damn sexy stroking himself. It definitely makes what is going to happen next pretty much a forgone conclusion.

'You're nearly done with the book then.'

I nod, dragging my eyes away from his cock to answer. 'Just a few bits left to tidy, here and there. I'm getting there.'

He stretches out slightly in the chair, making himself more comfortable, drawing my attention back to his lap, not that it needed much.

'So do you touch yourself when you write?'

Still focused on watching his hand move up and down I catch myself gnawing on my bottom lip in distraction and give myself a mental shake.

'No. If I'm writing something I usually know where I want it to go, so I'll take it there first, if the writing is flowing. If I'm writing about something that I find sexy then I might get aroused, but I won't do anything about it until I'm done.'

'That sounds frustrating.' I can hear the smile in his voice, although I'm still captivated by his cock rather than his face.

'It's not really. Since ultimately the release is within my control it doesn't feel such a hardship to wait if you feel like the writing's going OK, it's a trade off –' I tail off, hideously aware that I am now suffering from some form of verbal diarrhoea brought about because 95 per cent of my mind is thinking about the hot man wanking sat at my desk, leaving the final 5 per cent in charge of everything else.

'Is this bit about me?' My eyes flicker up to look at him, startled. 'Be honest.'

I look over his shoulder, see which chapter he's reading. I have to clear my throat before I can answer, embarrassed and also a bit on the back foot – mindful that with this book I have given him more of an insight into me, into how I see my relationship with him, than ever before. Wondering if this counts as being given enough rope to hang yourself. My voice is quiet and shy, which feels ridiculous when you think that I have spent the last six months spending a great part of my non-working hours writing some very smutty things indeed. 'Yes.'

His voice takes on the timbre which makes me wet and fearful at the same time. 'Get down on your knees.'

I don't move immediately. It's been a long week, and while this is fun and everything I'm not in the right headspace. Irony of ironies, I know, but I'm really not. Of course kneeling in front of him while he's sitting in the chair means I would have a really great view. *Sod it*, I think to myself and sink to the floor.

The thing is, I'm still crap at hiding anything. And being half-arsed about this stuff is just opening yourself up to trouble.

'You rolled your eyes then.'

'No I didn't.' Shit. Why the hell am I arguing? That was a mistake too. Shut up. Bugger it.

'Yes you did. And just then, that sounded like you answering back.'

I swear to God I am actually chewing on the words to argue that I wasn't answering back. I just about manage to keep them in but it's touch and go. And I'm fairly sure he can tell, although he looks more amused than pissed off. But then he's all back to business.

'Take your clothes off, except for your knickers, and get back down on your knees.'

My movements are quick and economical. This is no strip tease – I'm conscious I'm in quite enough trouble already so I obey quickly, keeping my gaze down as I drop to the floor so no real or imagined eye-rolling can get me into any more hot water.

His cock, hard and red and tempting, is just a few inches from my face, his hand still moving along it in mellow rhythm. My hands clench at my sides, with the effort of not moving to try and touch him.

'Pinch your nipples for me. Hard. Show me your tits. Come on.'

I start to pull and squeeze my nipples, lifting the weight of my breasts up. Being naked on display in front of him when he's fully dressed and looking like he's ready for a trip out for dinner is the kind of little humiliation he revels in and something, even now, I find difficult to deal with. I close my eyes at the embarrassment of it, can feel myself blushing a little, even as my knickers start feeling slick between my legs.

His hands slap mine away and he grabs and twists my nipples. My eyes open in shock and I can't stop a yelp at the pain, as he pulls my tits high, making me kneel higher to try and ease some of the tension.

'Your pinching is pathetic. This is what I mean.' He twists viciously to punctuate his point and I breathe deeply to try and process the wave of pain. 'Now do it properly. And look down, you don't even deserve to look at my cock at the moment.'

Now I don't know if this is something anyone else with submissive tendencies finds, but I am fine withstanding pain dished out by someone else – I'd even go so far as to say when I'm in the zone I have a fairly good tolerance for pain. But asking me to inflict it on myself? Somehow it's harder to withstand. Bearing in mind I can't wax my own legs because the thought of the pain leaves me incapable to rip the wax strips off. However, he's mightily pissed off now and so I twist my already red and sore nipples harder, eyes on the floor.

I honestly don't know how long we stay there. The room is still but for the movement of him stroking himself just outside of my peripheral vision. I am desperate to see him, but stare resolutely at a knot on the hard wood floor between his bare feet.

'It's a great view. I don't know where to come though. It seems a shame to come in your hair when you've just washed it. Maybe I should come across your tits. What do you think?'

I sneak a peek to see whether I'm supposed to reply, see him looking at me and am back staring at his toes before he finishes barking the command for me to look down. My voice is hesitant as I try and work out how to say I want him to come in my mouth. I love having him in my mouth. I love swallowing his spunk. But with my equilibrium off I feel uncertain the best way to say it and it ends up sounding like a question, which amuses him if nothing else.

Kneeling here in front of him staring at his feet, though, my mindset is shifting a gear. The weight of the week is easing, and all I'm aware of for now is how horny this gorgeous guy is making me and how desperate I am to please him so (and I know this isn't the point but forgive me for being self-indulgent) he'll please me. The idea of him touching me, letting me touch him is something I want so much that in this instant everything else is fading away.

'Stand up.'

I've been kneeling before him long enough that it takes me a couple of seconds to get my balance. He manoeuvres my shoulder so I'm facing the way he wants me to and then his fingers are sliding along my slit, pushing the slick cotton into my cunt and chuckling at how wet I am. I battle to stand still, looking straight ahead, as he runs his teasing fingers around my cunt and arse, stopping to draw a line down my spine which makes me shiver before pulling my knickers down. Thank fuck. I step out of them as they pool around my feet, and as I do so he grabs my hair, gathered in a ponytail at the nape of my neck, and pulls on it hard, yanking me to the floor in ungainly fashion. As I scramble to my knees he pulls me back against his hip bone, holding me in place.

'You're still doing things I've not asked you to do. I don't want you to show initiative. Right now, I don't want you to do anything but what I tell you to do when I tell you to do it. When I ask you a question you are to answer it promptly and politely. You're not unintelligent. These are simple things. Do you understand?'

My throat is dry. 'Yes. Sorry.'

The silence lengthens, me held in place by my hair, leaning against him while he stands over me like some kind of conquering hero.

'Right. You've not been anywhere near as obedient as you should have been today and you obviously still have much to learn despite how far you've come. How do you think I am going to teach you a lesson so you'll remember for next time?'

I know. God I know. But I don't want to be too specific in how I answer this in case I put ideas into his head. Is he wearing his belt today? Does he remember where I keep my toys?

He tugs on my hair. 'Well?'

'You're going to punish me.'

'Indeed.'

Once again I'm moving, manoeuvred into position leaning against the arm of the sofa. He kicks my legs open, so the slickness of my cunt is visible and then turns his attention to my arse, running his fingers along the sensitive curve of it, making me shiver while I wait for the first blow.

Now being on the receiving end of the cane and the belt at his hand have both reduced me to tears before. But when he's wanting to make an impression even a spanking can be painful. And as the sound of the first blow reverberates round the room and I suck air in through my teeth to ride the wave of pain I realise this is actual punishment, not some kind of play-acting spank session.

The thing is, as the blows rain down, and I hold my position, dealing with the pain clears everything else out of my head. I'm not thinking about my crappy week, not wondering about word counts and paragraph breaks, I'm not worrying what I look like naked with my arse in the air, I'm not even thinking about how horny I am (although, for the record, I am now desperate for him to allow me to come). I am just riding the waves of pain and withstanding the onslaught that he is dishing out, because at this point I know I need to do so, to take my punishment. My mind is clear and a weight has been lifted and all it has taken is a thorough thrashing of one arse cheek.

He stops for a second and asks how many times he has hit my arse. I can only guess, while trying not to tremble as he runs a finger along my now hot bottom. He makes me count off the second cheek, thanking him for every blow, and rest assured there is no eye-rolling by then, I'm too busy trying to stay upright and in position on wobbly legs.

Once he's finished he steps back and unceremoniously thrusts his fingers in my cunt from behind. Leaving me bent over in undignified fashion he puts an arm round my front to frig my clit and the onslaught has me whimpering and bucking beneath him like an animal as he fucks me with his fingers, being sure to bash the edge of my punished arse with his thumb during every thrust too. The sensation is intense. My cunt is sopping so he slips in and out of me easily, pushing me closer to orgasm, harder and harder while he rubs my clit so viciously that the intense pleasure is almost painful. Having stayed faithfully in position during the punishment, the pleasure is too much for me to stand and I end up coming hard on his fingers, sinking down to the floor where I huddle for a second trying to get my breath back. By definition, there's no such thing as a bad orgasm but this one is the perfect release at the end of the week. It's like I've been broken down and rebuilt.

As I become more aware of my surroundings, I lift myself up from my supine position on the floor to see him standing over me with his cock out. As he moves towards me, finally, I move my head towards him to take him in my mouth. But the sting in my scalp brings tears to my eyes as he pulls me back.

'You get my cock when I say you can have it.'

I open my mouth again, this time to apologise, but as I do he grabs the back of my head and shoves himself past my lips, leaving me struggling for a second to accept his cock without gagging. My mouth starts working on him, and I lick and suck him eagerly, enjoying feeling him thicken in my mouth, listening to his breathing change. At that moment the entire focus of my world is his cock and making sure I lick and suck him to his satisfaction. Nothing else matters and the simplicity of that feels exhilarating. As he spunks into my throat and I swallow his juice down I smile to myself and have a moment of contemplative peace.

Being submissive is just one facet of my personality. But it is a key part of what makes me the person I am: as much so as the importance I place on my friends and family, the way I love my job and the creativity and variety it brings me, my independent stubborn streak, my love of Marmite even.

Suddenly my shitty week, everything else that felt so urgent and important 20 minutes ago feels a world away. Right now, for this moment, my arse sore and the taste of his spunk in my throat, he is the centre of my universe. And I fucking love it.

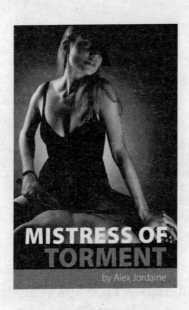

Mistress of Torment
Alex Jordaine

When dark fantasy turns to darkest reality…

Self-bondage addict Paul is submissive to the core but craves constant hard discipline. A chance meeting with an old friend brings him within the thrilling orbit of top professional dominatrix Mistress Nikki and the ultra-sadistic Mistress Alicia.

An erotic novel with strong BDSM and Femdom content.

ISBN 9781906373825, price £7.99

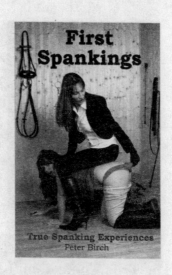

First Spankings – True Spanking Initiations
Peter Birch

Accounts of real spankings given to real women! From the occasional bit of fun to tales from the most dedicated enthusiasts, the detailed stories include well known names from the genre of spanking erotica, many personal friends of the author, and confessions from around the world. It's an enthusiast's book, no question, but if you're curious about what really makes the kinky girls tick, then this is a must for any erotica shelf.

Peter Birch has been spanking girls for thirty years now, and has collected stories from the thirties to the noughties. This is the very first encyclopaedic erotica collection of erotic punishment given by boys to girls, and given by girls to girls, even in public. And one thing is guaranteed: every single confession is a genuine account of a woman's first experience of going over the knee.

ISBN 9781907016271 price £7.99

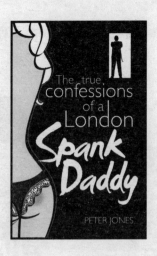

The True Confessions of a
London Spank Daddy
Peter Jones

Discover an underworld of sex, spanking and submission. A world where high-powered executives and cuddly mums go to be spanked, caned and disciplined.

In this powerful and compelling book Peter Jones reveals how his fetish was kindled by corporal punishment while still at school and how he struggled to contain it. Eventually, he discovered he was far from alone in London's vibrant, active sex scene.

Chapter by chapter he reveals his clients' stories as he turns their fantasies into reality. The writing is powerful, the stories graphic and compelling.

Discover an unknown world…

ISBN 9781906373320 Price £7.99

More Spanking Titles from Xcite Books

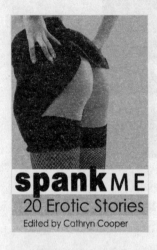

9781905170937 £7.99

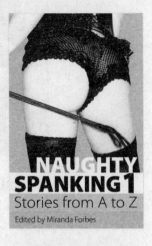

9781906125837 £7.99

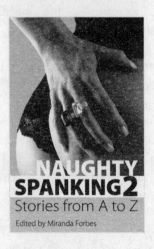

9781906125899 £7.99

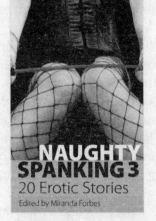

9781906373702 £7.99